ELEVENTH ED

The Joint Commission Survey Coordinator's Handbook

11

Patricia Pejakovich, RN, BSN, MPA, CPHQ

HCPro

The Joint Commission Survey Coordinator's Handbook, 11th Edition, is published by HCPro, Inc.

Copyright © 2009 HCPro, Inc. No claim to original U.S. government work.

All rights reserved. Printed in the United States of America.   5 4 3 2 1

ISBN 978-1-60146-704-1

No part of this publication may be reproduced, in any form or by any means, without prior written consent of HCPro, Inc., or the Copyright Clearance Center (978/750-8400). Please notify us immediately if you have received an unauthorized copy.

HCPro, Inc., provides information resources for the healthcare industry.

HCPro, Inc., is not affiliated in any way with The Joint Commission, which owns the JCAHO and Joint Commissions trademarks.

Patricia Pejakovich, RN, BSN, MPA, CPHQ, Author
Brad Keyes, CHSP, Contributing Author
Matt Phillion, Editor
Michael Briddon, Executive Editor
Emily Sheahan, Group Publisher
Amy Cohen, Proofreader

Susan Darbyshire, Cover Designer
Audrey Doyle, Copyeditor
Janell Lukac, Graphic Artist
Matt Sharpe, Production Supervisor
Jean St. Pierre, Director of Operations

Advice given is general. Readers should consult professional counsel for specific legal, ethical, or clinical questions.

Arrangements can be made for quantity discounts. For more information, contact:

HCPro, Inc.
P.O. Box 1168
Marblehead, MA 01945
Telephone: 800/650-6787 or 781/639-1872
Fax: 781/639-2982
E-mail: *customerservice@hcpro.com*

Visit HCPro at its World Wide Web sites:
www.hcpro.com **and** *www.hcmarketplace.com*

Contents

Figure List vi

About the Author viii

About the Contributor ix

Acknowledgments x

Chapter 1: The Joint Commission: An Overview 1
Why Seek Joint Commission Accreditation? 1
Accreditation Services 8
History of The Joint Commission 17
The Survey Process 36
Your Survey Team 43
Test Your Knowledge 44

Chapter 2: Addressing the Changes in Standards for 2009 45
Restraint and Seclusion 51
Noncompliance at a CMS Condition Level 60
Test Your Knowledge 65

Chapter 3: Frequently Cited Standards and How to Avoid Them 67
Issue 1: Failure to Check Crash Carts at the Frequency Required by the Organization's Policy 67
Issue 2: Pain Reassessments Not Performed in Accordance with Hospital Policy 69
Issue 3: Updated History and Physical on the Day of Surgery 74
Issue 4: Requiring an H&P Prior to Moderate Sedation 75
Issue 5: Untimely Primary Source Verification of Practitioner and Staff Licenses 76
Issue 6: Inadequate Monitoring of Contracted Clinical Services 79
Issue 7: Deviation from High-Level Disinfection Procedures 81
Issue 8: Missing or Incomplete Physician Orders 82

Chapter 4: Internally Assessing Standards Compliance 89
- Select an Approach to Self-Assessment 95
- Determine the Scoring Tool to Be Utilized 96
- It Takes a Team: Choose Participants Wisely 98
- Provide Education and Training to the Teams 99
- Document the Evidence of Compliance 102
- Assessment versus "Parking Lot" Issues 103
- Categorize the Noncompliant Findings for Action 103
- Report the Initial Results to Key Stakeholders 104
- Begin the Improvement Process 105
- Why Do Internal Assessments Sometimes Fail? 107
- Sustaining Compliance 108
- Test Your Knowledge 114

Chapter 5: *Life Safety Code* Compliance for the Nonengineer 115
- The *Statement of Conditions* (LS.01.01.01) 115
- Interim Life Safety Measures (LS.01.02.01) 117
- Minimizing the Effects of Fire and Smoke (LS.02.01.10) 118
- Means of Egress (LS.02.01.20) 118
- Protection from Hazards of Fire and Smoke (LS.02.01.30) 121
- Fire Alarm Systems and Sprinkler Systems (LS.02.01.34 and LS.02.01.35) 123
- Building Services and Operating Features (LS.02.01.50 and LS.02.01.70) 125
- In Conclusion 126
- Test Your Knowledge 128

Chapter 6: The National Patient Safety Goals 129
- Moved NPSGs 130
- Deleted NPSGs 132
- A Closer Look at Some of the Revisions for 2010 132
- Survey Emphasis on NPSGs 144
- Test Your Knowledge 146

Chapter 7: Ready, Set, Survey: Methods for Preparing for and Managing Your Survey 147

    References for Planning 148

    Focus on the Front End, and Plan Carefully 149

    Define Expected Responses Following Survey Notification 163

    Practice Your Plan 166

    Day of Survey 170

    Exit Briefing 172

    Test Your Knowledge 173

Chapter 8: The Challenges of Required Written Documentation 175

    The Required Documents: One by One 179

    Medical Staff Credentialing and Privileging 187

    Test Your Knowledge 191

Chapter 9: After-Survey Activities 193

    The Next Step: Identifying Opportunities for Clarification 194

    Evaluating the Success of the Organization's Unannounced Survey Plan 201

    Maintain Survey Readiness 202

    Identify Methods to Monitor Standards Compliance 203

    Test Your Knowledge 209

Appendix: Additional Forms 211

Figure List

Figure 2.1	Hospitalwide Performance Improvement Annual Workplan	63
Figure 2.2	Letter for Completion of Grievance Investigation	64
Figure 3.1	Pain Assessment Tools	72
Figure 3.2	Contracted Clinical Services Checklist	80
Figure 4.1	Gap Analysis	91
Figure 4.2	Gap Analysis Documentation	92
Figure 4.3	Data Collection Worksheet	101
Figure 4.4	TJC Continuous Survey Readiness Action Plan	106
Figure 4.5	You've Been Traced	111
Figure 5.1	Requirements for Portable Fire Extinguishers	124
Figure 6.1	Hospital NPSG 2010 Retained	130
Figure 6.2	Hospital NPSG 2010 Moved as of October 29, 2009	131
Figure 7.1	Checklist for Unannounced Joint Commission Survey Plan	150
Figure 7.2	Sample Fact Sheet	159
Figure 7.3	Survey Activities	160
Figure 7.4	Surveyor Escort Duties	161
Figure 7.5	Typical Command Center Duties	162
Figure 7.6	Sample Phone Log	165
Figure 7.7	Greeters' Duties	167
Figure 7.8	Escort Documentation Worksheet	169
Figure 8.1	Information Management Circle D Elements of Performance	176

Appendix

Figure A.1	"Show Me" Tracer—Most Challenging Standards	212
Figure A.2	Labeling of Secondary Containers	216
Figure A.3	Improving Patient Identification	217
Figure A.4	Patient Reporting of Safety Concerns	218
Figure A.5	Guidelines for Surgical/Procedural Documentation Requirements	219
Figure A.6	Determining Patient Restraint or Seclusion	222

Figure A.7 ■ Joint Commission Survey Individual Tracer Unit Survey Sheet 223

Figure A.8 ■ OB Vaginal Delivery—Tracer Recording Form 224

Figure A.9 ■ OB Cesarean Section—Tracer Recording Form 226

Figure A.10 ■ Infection Control—Tracer Recording Form 227

Figure A.11 ■ Emergency Department—Tracer Recording Form 228

Figure A.12 ■ Resource Web Sites 230

> **All of the figures located or referenced in the body of this book as well as the appendix are available online at *www.hcpro.com/downloads/8088*.**
> Please note: Bonus materials not appearing in this book also appear in the appendix free to download with the purchase of this book.

About the Author

Patricia Pejakovich, RN, BSN, MPA, CPHQ

Ms. Pejakovich is a senior consultant with The Greeley Company. She brings over 25 years of management experience to her work with healthcare organizations across the nation.

Ms. Pejakovich applies leadership and nursing experiences to help hospitals and medical staffs develop solutions to their toughest problems. She has a particular expertise in accreditation standards and regulatory compliance. Ms. Pejakovich has consulted on utilization management, credentialing, data management and design, hospital and medical staff quality improvement processes, forms, documents, tools and reports to support improvement activities, infection control, organizational readiness for survey, policy and procedure development, and employee orientation and competency assessments.

In her role of senior consultant, Ms. Pejakovich has authored *The Joint Commission Survey Coordinator's Handbook,* Ninth Edition, *Tracer Methodology,* 2nd Edition, and *The Foundation of Patient Care.*

Prior to joining The Greeley Company, Ms. Pejakovich worked 15 years in hospital senior management with responsibility for quality improvement, medical staff credentialing, continuing medical education, infection control, case management, JCAHO accreditation, and data abstracting. She also served as corporate director of quality improvement for a large HMO and with a state medical society assisting physicians in negotiating third-party payer contracts.

Ms. Pejakovich holds an M.S. in public administration/healthcare from Western Michigan University. She received a B.S. in nursing from the University of Michigan.

Ms. Pejakovich maintains memberships with the National Association for Healthcare Quality and Michigan Association for Healthcare Quality.

About the Contributor

Brad Keyes, CHSP

Mr. Keyes (Chapter 5) is a safety engineer and consultant to healthcare organizations and a consultant with The Greeley Company. His expertise lies in the management of the Environment of Care, development of leadership effectiveness, and efficiency in work processes. This work focuses on life safety issues, assessing an organization's preparedness for survey, evaluating processes in achieving preparedness, and guiding organizations toward compliance.

Mr. Keyes' clients have included insurance underwriter groups, hospitals, ambulatory care centers, and large integrated systems across the country. He has been effective in training large groups as well as meeting one-on-one with healthcare leaders. This work has involved organizational assessment; management training; the ongoing coaching of task groups; and extensive, one-on-one coaching of facility leaders. He presents at national seminars and audio conferences.

Prior to joining The Greeley Company, Mr. Keyes has worked in the healthcare field in different capacities for over 30 years, most recently in the position of safety officer for a large Midwest hospital. He also was one of the original *Life Safety Code*® specialist surveyors for The Joint Commission and has over three years of experience with hospital accreditation surveys.

Mr. Keyes has published a variety of articles addressing features of healthcare fire protection and of the Building Maintenance Program. He is certified as a healthcare safety professional by the Board of Certified Healthcare Safety Management.

Acknowledgments

A heartfelt thank you to the very special contributors to this book.

Brad Keyes, CHSP, your chapter (Chapter 5) is so helpful to those of us who do not know a suite of rooms from a hotel suite. Thank you for writing such a useful and understandable chapter for our readers.

Wendy Sue Woods, RN, MHSA, senior consultant with The Greeley Company, we appreciate your article on policies. It was enlightening and addressed a hot topic still on our tables today.

Gayle Bielanski, RN, BS, consultant with The Greeley Company, helped simplify a complex subject and provided us with insights on what is required with the revised standards (included in the online appendix with this book). Thanks, Gayle, for authoring an informative article regarding restraints.

Unique educational tools called "Joint Points" were developed by **Lisa Eddy, RN, BSN,** senior consultant with The Greeley Company. These tools are eye-catching and true to their name—are "right to the point" when it comes to teaching the Joint Commission requirements to a multidisciplinary audience. Thanks, Lisa, for sharing these wonderful tools.

A special thank you to **Janelle Holth, RN, BSN,** regulatory compliance coordinator and **Jodi Sorum, MSW,** patient safety coordinator at Altru Health System in Grand Forks, ND, for sharing their unique "Show Me" tracer. Readers should find this user-friendly form helpful in their quest to assess implementation of standards and National Patient Safety Goals (included in the the back of this book).

Jason Miller, MPH, director of accreditation at Arkansas Children's Hospital in Little Rock, has graciously shared a flowchart of the restraint process he developed. Thanks to Jason, anyone who learns through visuals will find the numerical decision points extremely informative (please find this tool in the appendix section of this book).

Jodi L. Eisenberg, MHA, CPHQ, CPMSM, CSHA, program manager, accreditation and clinical compliance at Northwestern Memorial Hospital in Chicago, agreed to share her detailed spreadsheet prepared to assist staff in identifying the "D" elements of performance required for each chapter. Added columns in the spreadsheet are included for recording your organization's policy and the most recent update. An excellent addition to any accreditation specialist's toolbox (included in the online tools library included with this book).

Multiple forms for survey preparation were provided by **Jean Clark, RHIA, CSHA,** director of health information services at Roper St. Francis Health Services in Charleston, SC. An important aspect of a successful survey is coordinating the command center and selecting surveyor escorts who are judicial in recording tracer activities. Thanks to Jean's generosity, we have some forms that are survey ready (Chapter 8).

And to **Matt Phillion,** the most patient editor at HCPro, thanks for urging me to complete this book. Your diligence in deciphering my crazy late-night edits is remarkable. It is your skill of converting my words to readable text that makes this book a better product for the reader.

CHAPTER 1

The Joint Commission: An Overview

This chapter will help you, the accreditation specialist, to understand how The Joint Commission has evolved over time and how some of the changes have led to frustrations among hospital personnel and medical staff members. In addition, it will provide you with some tips on how you might approach changes as they continue to occur. For those who are unfamiliar with the scope of The Joint Commission, the chapter also provides an overview of the organization's multiple accreditation and certification programs and includes a reference to each program's Web site for obtaining additional information.

Some of the activities within the survey process, such as the tracer methodology and system tracers, will be described, as well as survey "dos and don'ts" that I have learned in the past few years. This chapter provides you with an overview of the basics of The Joint Commission and is intended to supplement or summarize the information found in standards manuals.

Why Seek Joint Commission Accreditation?

Today, The Joint Commission accredits more than 16,000 healthcare programs in organizations throughout the United States. Of those programs, 4,245 are hospitals. This means that The Joint Commission has accredited approximately 88% of the nation's hospitals. The Joint Commission is currently one of three entities with "deemed status" from the Centers for Medicare & Medicaid Services (CMS) that a hospital may select for accreditation.

Chapter 1

Although accreditation is not required by law, not having accreditation puts healthcare facilities at a disadvantage in terms of public image, competitiveness, and the capability to borrow money or float bond issues. But perhaps one of the most important issues to hospital operations is the deemed status with CMS that allows facilities to participate in Medicaid and Medicare as a third-party payer.

> **Key Concept**
>
>
>
> Even though your facility is accredited by The Joint Commission, this does not mean your state surveyors will not arrive at your facility to conduct a CMS survey, follow up on a complaint, or evaluate state licensing regulations. And although this book is focused on The Joint Commission, the principles it outlines are applicable to both CMS and state licensing surveys.

Without acquiring accreditation from The Joint Commission or from the Healthcare Facilities Accreditation Program (HFAP) operated by the American Osteopathic Association (AOA) or, most recently, approved by DNV Healthcare, Inc., hospitals would not be eligible to bill Medicare and Medicaid. According to the payer mix of many hospitals, most patient care revenue comes from Medicare and Medicaid payments. Thus, removal from those programs would have a major negative effect on a hospital's bottom line.

Washington Hospital Switches to DNV Accreditation

For one Washington hospital, making the move from Joint Commission accreditation to DNV Healthcare, Inc.'s NIAHO accreditation was a matter of research, timing ... and moving at a lightning pace.

Group Health Central Hospital is part of Group Health Cooperative, an integrated delivery and financing system providing care to approximately 400,000 residents of Washington and Northern Idaho. The organization operates 26 primary care centers, three specialty centers, and one hospital.

"It all started out at the annual Institute for Healthcare Improvement National Forum," says **Elizabeth Rosen, RN, BSN,** director of quality and regulatory compliance for Central Hospital. "DNV was there, and I discussed the situation with them and came back to share my interest with our leadership."

The hospital's chief of hospital medical staff, director of clinical operations, and Rosen met with DNV to determine whether the change was worth pursuing. Next, they brought in hospital administration, the chief nursing officer, the vice president of acute care, and legal counsel.

"I had outlined a proposal with a comparison of the Joint Commission and NIAHO standards," says Rosen. "People were all positive, though there was some concern about the time frame."

And what a time frame it was. The hospital was due anytime after January 1 for a Joint Commission survey. Regardless of whether it was changing accrediting organizations, Group Health was subject to the survey and could not change accrediting organizations if it had any outstanding requirements for improvement with the old accrediting organization.

The decision went from hospital leadership to the CEO of the overall organization.

"The CEO, in consultation with the board of trustees, made the final decision," says Rosen. "At the same time this decision-making process was going on, we did a high-level gap analysis to look at the differences between DNV and The Joint Commission, to understand where our focus areas would be."

> **Washington Hospital Switches to DNV Accreditation (Cont.)**
>
> The hospital's legal counsel reviewed the contract template, and the application was filled out during the decision-making process because everyone involved knew the change would have to happen fast.
>
> "We made the final decision to withdraw from The Joint Commission, and immediately following withdrawal sent our application to DNV," says Rosen.
>
> After signing the contract, the hospital began working with DNV to establish a timeline for the survey process—all in all, about a month elapsed between the signing of the contract and the arrival of DNV surveyors.
>
> "We had to move very quickly," says **Mary Lou Calise, RN, BS, MSQA, CPHQ,** quality consultant for Group Health. "We needed to be very compliant in a very short time period."
>
> Given how closely aligned the NIAHO standards are to CMS regulations, Calise says they were "pleasantly surprised during this process."
>
> Because there would be a time gap between Joint Commission and DNV accreditation, Rosen worked with the state Department of Health and the local CMS office to keep it up to speed regarding the hospital's accreditation status.
>
> **Pros and Cons**
>
> Group Health made its decision after weighing the upsides and downsides to both accrediting bodies.
>
> "We went over the pros and cons," says Rosen. "Central Hospital is a very limited hospital—we'd previously had two hospitals [in the system], but closed one in 2008 as part of an affiliation with an existing tertiary community hospital, so we went from a hospital system with a number of regular inpatient/acute care units to having obstetrics inpatient with all other hospital-based outpatient units."
>
> One of the issues Group Health was having concerned the inpatient-oriented approach of the Joint Commission's standards, which no longer made sense based on how Group Health's services had changed with the closing of the second hospital.

Washington Hospital Switches to DNV Accreditation (Cont.)

"This was the biggest reason for changing," says Rosen. "Another was that, especially in 2008 and 2009, the Joint Commission standards were becoming so prescriptive that it wasn't fitting with our services and population."

The frequency and volume of the Joint Commission's changes were difficult on small hospitals, says Rosen.

"Some of the standards wouldn't apply to us or [would] have [a] limited result on our population," says Rosen. "Instead, [now] we're able to focus our energies with more applicability."

For example, the hospital has only a very small number of overnight patients requiring anticoagulant management. A process for managing these patients has been put into place and the hospital stands behind it, but it might not have been a priority focus area given the hospital's patient needs.

"What I looked at was the NIAHO standards in comparison with what was currently being done at our facility for compliance," says Calise.

She worked to marry the two sets of requirements, looking for weaknesses and for areas where the facility needed to change course or stay on course. It was very site-specific.

"For example, CMS has extended their restraints standards," says Calise. "We were in compliance, but we don't have a psychiatric unit. We use restraints very infrequently. We had to take a closer look at what we were doing and where we needed to go."

Timing of Surveys

Also in the plus column: annual surveys.

"We saw a benefit to an annual survey," which DNV requires, says Rosen. The upside of this frequency would be "having some sense of when you can anticipate when the survey would be and also keeping on top of everything all the time," she says.

Calise agrees.

> **Washington Hospital Switches to DNV Accreditation (Cont.)**
>
> "Coming once a year ... those of us working in quality are all for it," she says. DNV offers to train one person in the facility to be a surveyor—the facility pays for travel expenses, and this designee must survey three other facilities each year. He or she is also trained in ISO 9001 compliance.
>
> "We liked the idea of a collaborative approach," says Rosen. "We liked the idea of having one of our own internal quality folks become a DNV surveyor and becoming our in-house expert."
>
> That person, in Group Health's case, will be Calise.
>
> "I used to be a surveyor for the Commission on Accreditation of Rehabilitation Facilities," says Calise. "When I'd see a different way of doing something well, I'd bring that knowledge back to my facility. You're always learning, finding different ways to accomplish your goals."
>
> Calise is looking forward to the challenges NIAHO certification will provide.
>
> "I'm very pro-data, and this is looking at your data, doing an analysis of it, and looking for where the faults are [and] tweaking it to get your system where it needs to be," says Calise.
>
> Another selling point for Group Health was the concept of "no tipping point" for findings, says Rosen. Hospitals are instead required to have a corrective action plan in place and meet the time frames established for that plan.
>
> "I can't deny [that] I didn't understand the scoring system for The Joint Commission," says Rosen. "You didn't really know if there was a tipping point with the new [2009] scoring."
>
> **Leaving The Joint Commission**
>
> After submitting the withdrawal notice, the Group Health hospital administrator received a call from the Joint Commission account representative to schedule an exit interview.
>
> "Toward the end of the interview, they wanted to know the actual date of withdrawal," says Rosen. The letter had said "immediately." Whatever date is specified for the withdrawal, The Joint Commission sends a notification to CMS to say the facility is no longer subject to Joint Commission accreditation. It was unclear what implications, if any, the notice to CMS might have concerning the hospital's continuing Medicare certification.

Washington Hospital Switches to DNV Accreditation (Cont.)

"Our understanding was that our [Joint Commission accreditation] certificate was effective through mid-March 2009," says Rosen.

According to the Joint Commission representative, however, the minute you withdraw you go into nonaccreditation status, Rosen says. This left the hospital in a quandary: If you do not withdraw immediately, you are still subject to a Joint Commission survey at any time, even if the hospital is in the process of changing to a different accreditation body.

"We were a little surprised at that," says Rosen. "So we reviewed the situation with our attorney and with our accreditation consultant at The Greeley Company and were assured it was not a significant issue."

Coincidentally, a week after the DNV survey is scheduled, the hospital will undergo its regular state licensing survey. Under current Washington state law, the state's Department of Health is required to conduct periodic hospital surveys, but may forego conducting a survey during a year in which a hospital is surveyed by The Joint Commission or by the AOA. The law reflects the fact that for more than 30 years, The Joint Commission and the AOA had been the only hospital accreditation entities approved by CMS. This changed in fall 2008, when CMS approved DNV Healthcare as another option for achieving deemed status under Medicare.

"Because the state of Washington has not yet added DNV as an option, we still need to have a licensing survey," says Rosen. Group Health is working closely with the Washington State Hospital Association and the Department of Health to change the law and recognize DNV for purposes of future state surveys.

Once NIAHO accreditation has been achieved, the next step will be to implement the second component to DNV accreditation: use of ISO 9001.

"ISO 9001 is centered [on] quality," says Calise. "Industry has been doing it for a long time. It's looking at processes, making sure you're meeting the standards you're reaching for, and if not, adjusting them to make sure you do."

Source: **Briefings on The Joint Commission,** April 2009.

Note: If you are unfamiliar with HFAP, log on to *www.hfap.org* to learn more about its accreditation program. The Web site for DNV is *www.dnv.com/focus/hospital_accreditation.*

Joint Commission accreditation benefits your hospital financially, but compliance with the Joint Commission's standards also can help fulfill the most important objective of all: providing safe, quality patient care. As an accreditation specialist, have you often wondered how many hospitals would actually seek accreditation if the financial component was not a pressing issue? Indeed, to comply with the Joint Commission standards, hospital leaders and staff members must be knowledgeable of the requirements, integrate standards into daily operations, and be willing to revise processes as needed while continuing to provide high-quality and safe services.

Although continuously preparing for a Joint Commission survey can be time-consuming, labor-intensive, and expensive, hospitals should seek to recognize the value that accreditation brings to the organization. With a few exceptions, the Joint Commission standards are operationally sound and focused on the delivery of patient care that keeps the patient safe and improves the patient's healthcare experience. People who cannot support such objectives might want to seriously ask themselves why they are working in healthcare.

Accreditation Services

In addition to general hospitals, The Joint Commission currently provides accreditation services to a multitude of other healthcare organizations listed in this section.

A complex hospital, defined as a hospital that uses more than one manual in its survey process and is governed by the Tailored Survey Policy, may elect to have separate surveys for its ambulatory, home care, long-term care, or behavioral services. In this scenario, each service stands alone for the count of Requirements for Improvement (RFI) findings and meeting the program-specific "bands" to determine the number of noncompliant direct impacts an organization may receive before being reviewed by the Joint Commission's central office.

Each Web site listed in parentheses in the following sections takes you to a Web page with information specific to that program. I am providing this list in case you are a new accreditation specialist and are not aware of the extent of accreditation services that The Joint Commission provides.

Ambulatory care services

This includes outpatient surgery centers, rehabilitation facilities, infusion centers, group practices, sleep labs, imaging centers, community health centers, and other outpatient services. As of 2004, the Accreditation Council for Graduate Medical Education requires university medical schools that provide clinical services to obtain ambulatory accreditation. If your organization is utilizing a radiology group for telemedicine, perhaps it is accredited by The Joint Commission. If so, this would be the accreditation for that type of service.

(www.jointcommission.org/AccreditationPrograms/AmbulatoryCare)

Behavioral healthcare organizations

This includes organizations offering the following services for patients: mental health services, treatment for chemical dependency, and mental retardation/development disabilities services. More than 1,800 behavioral health organizations have sought this accreditation.

Note: Acute care hospitals with a behavioral health unit may choose to use this accreditation program in addition to the hospital standards.

(www.jointcommission.org/AccreditationPrograms/BehavioralHealthCare)

Clinical laboratories

Nearly 2,000 organizations with laboratory services, including freestanding laboratories and those connected with other healthcare organizations, are accredited by The Joint Commission. Many of you may be familiar only with CAP accreditation from the College of American Pathologists, but The Joint Commission is an alternative.

(www.jointcommission.org/AccreditationPrograms/LaboratoryServices)

Critical access hospitals

These are hospitals that have a census of fewer than 25 patients and are located more than 35 miles from a hospital or another critical access hospital. A hospital certified by its state as necessary to provide healthcare services to residents in the area is also considered a critical access hospital. The critical access standards vary somewhat from the hospital standards, so read carefully to identify those nuances.

(www.jointcommission.org/AccreditationPrograms/CriticalAccessHospitals)

Home care organizations

This includes organizations offering home health services, personal care and support services, home infusion and pharmacy services, durable medical equipment, and hospice services. More than 4,000 entities are accredited by The Joint Commission.

(www.jointcommission.org/AccreditationPrograms/HomeCare)

Long-term care

This includes nursing home facilities, including dementia programs, subacute programs, and long-term care pharmacies. The Joint Commission has been accrediting these organizations—more than 1,100 of them—for more than 40 years.

(www.jointcommission.org/AccreditationPrograms/LongTermCare)

Office-based surgery centers

The Joint Commission accredits more than 400 outpatient settings, including oral surgeons, endoscopy suites, plastic surgery practices, and laser surgery clinics.

(www.jointcommission.org/AccreditationPrograms/Office-BasedSurgery)

International accreditation

Launched in 1999, The Joint Commission's international accreditation program has been growing over the past several years and, at the time of this writing, accredits organizations in more than 20 countries. This program accredits international healthcare organizations, including hospitals, ambulatory facilities, laboratories, medical transport agencies, public health agencies, and health ministries.

The Joint Commission's international standards are based on international consensus standards, and the process is designed to meet legal, religious, and cultural factors. As a way to help build a more global presence, in recent years the organization developed The Joint Commission International Center for Patient Safety, a Web resource with links to a best-practices database and other helpful information for domestic or international organizations to maintain their accreditation.

Certification services and disease-specific care

More recently, The Joint Commission began offering a variety of certification programs. At the time of this writing, the Joint Commission Web site listed seven advance certifications and 29 disease-specific certifications. An organization does not have to be Joint Commission–accredited to apply for a certification, but many Joint Commission–accredited organizations opt for certification in service areas, such as stroke. Following are the certification programs:

- Acute coronary syndrome
- Alzheimer's disease
- Arthritis
- Asthma
- Cancer
- Chronic kidney disease (in partnership with the National Kidney Foundation)
- Chronic obstructive pulmonary disease (COPD)
- Congestive heart failure
- Coronary artery disease
- Depression
- Diabetes
- Emphysema
- Epilepsy
- Healthcare staffing services (an evaluation of an organization's staffing practices, such as verifying credentials and competencies of the healthcare staff)
- Hemophilia
- High-risk pregnancy
- HIV/AIDS
- Hypertension
- Inpatient diabetes (new in 2006, this applies to organizations with patients who have a medical history of diabetes diagnosed and acknowledged by a treating physician)
- Ischemic heart disease
- Low back pain
- Lung volume reduction surgery (for hospitals performing this procedure)

- Migraines

- Multiple sclerosis

- Obesity/bariatric surgery

- Osteoporosis

- Parkinson's disease

- Primary stroke (in partnership with the American Stroke Association)

- Sickle cell disease

- Transplant center (this program was under development in 2006)

- Ventricular assist device or VAD (for hospitals performing VAD as a destination therapy)

When Multiple Disease-Specific Care Surveys Arrive

On the upside, disease-specific care (DSC) certification surveys provide a little more notice for hospitals than triennials, because The Joint Commission announces surveys six to eight weeks in advance rather than arriving unannounced. On the downside, in a six-hospital system with multiple DSC programs, those surveys can arrive uncomfortably close together.

"Disease-specific care has been functioning for many years, and it acts as a mark of excellence," says **Elizabeth Di Giacomo-Geffers, RN, MPH, CSHA,** a healthcare consultant in Trabuco Canyon, CA, and former Joint Commission surveyor.

For Main Line Health, a six-hospital system outside Bryn Mawr, PA, this meant four surveys in three hospitals from February 2009 through August 2009. With the right prep work, however, four surveys in a six-month period did not necessitate wide-scale panic, says **Mary McKay, RN, MS, CPHQ,** system director of regulatory affairs and nursing quality. The system weathered a VAD destination therapy program, primary stroke center certification, and two knee and hip programs successfully in a matter of weeks.

The prep work for a DSC survey is similar to preparations for The Joint Commission's triennial survey, says McKay.

When Multiple Disease-Specific Care Surveys Arrive (Cont.)

"It's very similar—you do your annual periodic performance review (PPR) and take your action plan from that," says McKay.

Main Line Health is also part of the Continual Survey Readiness program, which provides a self-assessment similar to the PPR. Each program underwent a self-assessment, devised action plans, and brought in clinical leaders to help push for improvements.

"With these certifications, the closer you get to the clinical area, the more robust the program is going to be—you'll have a better sustainability and compliance," says McKay.

In the weeks leading into the surveys, mock surveys were conducted either internally or through a consultant.

"Six to eight weeks before the survey we have our own internal tracers we conduct, focusing on those areas impacted by the program," says McKay.

Stay vigilant in all areas before the surveyors arrive, she says.

"One caution—don't ignore the rest of the patients or the rest of the unit," says McKay. "You know they're coming in to survey you for stroke or knee and hip, but it's still important that all of your admission assessments are complete. Nutritional, pain screening, falls ... they want to know you're addressing patient safety. Don't lose sight of those."

Surprises
McKay found that surveyors were very interested in education during DSC surveys.

"One quote all of the surveyors used [was] 'What makes you different?' " she says. " 'What sets you apart from the hospital down the street?' That's a message we hadn't seen in print before, and it really drove the message home, to refine the program and give it a unique look."

In addition, McKay found that the education component is more prescriptive in some programs than others.

When Multiple Disease-Specific Care Surveys Arrive (Cont.)

"With stroke, there's a big education requirement," says McKay. "Each staff [member] was asked, whether they were nursing or therapy or anyone else, what additional training [they] had in this area. And whether you're looking at stroke, or knee and hip, or VAD, that education sets you apart."

Staff education also reflects on the hospital as a whole.

"From the surveyor's point of view, they also want to know that having this additional education shows leadership's commitment to the program. Education is part of the organization's goals," says McKay.

For its knee and hip certification program, the healthcare organization had developed an individual care plan for patient education.

"Folks come in with a preop visit, and that education follows them through their hospital stay," says McKay. "Post-discharge there's a chance to participate in further education."

The organization was able to demonstrate the content and initial education to the knee and hip patient and document the patient's understanding, which reflected well on the program during the survey.

Patient education was one area in which the stroke program received an RFI—in this case, it wasn't that the education was not being provided, but simply had to do with documentation of such education.

"We use nursing pathways, and we haven't gone fully electronic yet," says McKay. "Because we use prepopulated pathways, they were not specific enough for stroke education."

Although the surveyor saw and believed that the facility was performing the appropriate level of education, the generic template for documenting this education will be improved.

That being said, the programs performed remarkably well during the surveys. Two of the four programs came away without a single RFI, and the other two programs had only two findings each.

When Multiple Disease-Specific Care Surveys Arrive (Cont.)

A lot of the success of these surveys came from the excellence of Main Line's staff education component.

"I have to give kudos to our nursing staff educators," says McKay. "I think the challenge will be in sustaining this going forward, always remembering [that] this population of the staff needs more than the mandatory training sessions. We need to give them refreshers in joints, VAD, [and] stroke."

Recertification

The second time around should be a very different experience, says McKay. "I'm looking forward to the recertifications," she says. "I think in some ways, as we know now what to expect, they'll be easier."

Main Line has already begun to identify areas that will be a challenge prior to the next round of surveys. First will be tracking standards as they change—the "unknown" factor between surveys, McKay says.

Also, tracking new staff members and the necessary education will be pivotal.

"As you acquire new staff [members], you have to have process(es) to capture their data, [and] put them into the pipeline for ongoing training and education," says McKay.

A number of unexpected points came up before, during, and after the survey:

- **Clinical competencies:** "For these units, they need particular competencies that are going to speak to how they are competent; what sets them apart from nurses on an adjacent floor," says McKay.

- **Older competency policies:** "Our competencies were age-specific, which are passé," says McKay. "We are moving to population-based." Although the system has done well on past surveys, they know that, having gone through four DSCs, the competencies will need to be updated for the next triennial survey and for DSC recertifications.

When Multiple Disease-Specific Care Surveys Arrive (Cont.)

- **HR files:** "We were surprised at the number of HR files they pulled," says McKay. Or rather, the lack thereof: For each survey, fewer than five HR files were requested.

How do they compare?

The surveyors were extremely personable, says McKay, and they offered a great deal of guidance and education, leaving behind helpful tools for improving processes.

"We have that sort of back and forth during the triennial, but there's a more personal aspect to the DSC surveys," she says.

With a single surveyor, a professional bond forms more quickly, McKay says.

In terms of workload, the more focused nature of a DSC survey—although intense—is in many ways more manageable. Issues that arise tend to be program-specific and not systemwide.

Systemwide issues can occur, however. For instance, in 2008, The Joint Commission changed its standard for primary source verification. Even if a hospital changed its process, it needs to verify that such a change is implemented correctly and sustained. If even one clerk does not implement the change and continues to operate under the old standard, this can impact the whole system when it comes time for any survey, DSC or triennial.

What's next?

Main Line Health is not done with its DSC surveys yet. The remaining facilities are still in the process of setting up initial certification for knee and hip programs, stroke, and COPD in the next six to nine months.

After that, they will be looking at the first rounds of recertifications.

"With recertification, they give you a window," says McKay. "In the second year, you have five days' advance notice of the survey. It's enough to make sure people are there and to get the appropriate materials ready, but not enough to perfect everything if you're not already ready for survey."

Source: **Briefings on The Joint Commission,** June 2009.

History of The Joint Commission

It is important that accreditation specialists understand the evolution of The Joint Commission. It didn't just spring up to make us struggle with compliance issues. It began almost 100 years ago and was based on the assessment of patient care. As you read the history, think about the impact on senior physicians and hospital staff members who have experienced the multitude of changes the accreditation process has gone through over the years.

In 1910, Ernest Codman, MD, proposed that hospitals develop procedures for tracking patients long enough to determine whether treatment was effective. By reviewing these outcomes, hospitals could evaluate their processes and procedures to gauge whether they needed to make improvements.

His innovative thinking resulted in a forced separation of practice from the esteemed Massachusetts General Hospital. Yet Codman's methods caught the attention of the American College of Surgeons (ACS), an organization founded in 1913, and the methods became part of the ACS' stated objectives. The ACS also used Codman's ideas to develop the "Minimum Standards for Hospitals," a short list of requirements designed to regulate quality of care. In 1918, the ACS used this list to begin its first on-site inspection of hospitals. The inspection program was so successful that, by 1950, more than 3,200 hospitals had earned the ACS' "seal of approval."

Codman's original documents remain stored in a vault, and a replica of his recommended processes is on display in the Center for Quality and Patient Safety at, ironically, Massachusetts General Hospital. Today, The Joint Commission continues to annually present the Ernest Amory Codman Award to recognize excellence in performance measurement.

In 1951, the ACS joined with the American College of Physicians, the American Hospital Association, the American Medical Association, and the Canadian Medical Association (CMA) to create The Joint Commission on Accreditation of Hospitals (JCAH). In 1959, the CMA withdrew to form its own Canadian accreditation organization. An independent, nonprofit organization, the JCAH provided voluntary accreditation to hospitals beginning in January 1953.

The JCAH received its deemed status soon after, in the 1960s, when the federal government created the Medicare program. The government decided that if it was going to pay hospitals for the care given to entitled patients, it needed a way to ensure that the quality of care at those hospitals warranted payment. The sponsoring federal agency in charge of Medicare realized that it did not have the resources, personnel, or expertise to conduct evaluations.

In response to this dilemma, in 1965 Congress passed the Medicare Act. The legislation states that hospitals accredited by the JCAH would be "deemed" to be in compliance with most of the Medicare *Conditions of Participation (CoP)* for hospitals.

As previously stated, *CoPs* are the minimum requirements hospitals still have to meet today to qualify for reimbursement from Medicare and Medicaid. With the passage of this act, the JCAH, a private organization, became an official inspection agency, and a Joint Commission survey was more like an audit than the educational experience it is today. Surveyors reviewed documents to determine whether policies and procedures were acceptable, whether people attended meetings, whether the organization addressed clinical problems, and whether top managers were competent. They also focused heavily on the safety and physical structure of hospital facilities.

To provide some insight on the impact of The Joint Commission to practicing physicians, please see the following excerpt from the HCPro publication *The Greeley Guide to New Medical Staff Models:*

> *During the 1970s, The Joint Commission began to require medical staffs to perform audits to measure the performance of their peers. Such a change was a direct threat to the clublike culture of most medical staffs, creating the potential for conflicts among physicians. Up to that point, even morbidity and mortality conferences had been confidential, undocumented discussions. Writing down the results of a case review, assigning it a score, and conducting other audit activities was anathema to most physicians. This created the first crack in the organized medical staff culture as it had developed.*

In 1987, the JCAH changed its name to The Joint Commission on the Accreditation of Healthcare Organizations, or JCAHO, to better reflect the changing scope of its services and the organizations that it surveyed. The standards were department-specific rather than cross-disciplinary, and they were organized by clinical department in the *Accreditation Manual for Hospitals (AMH)*, which listed Joint Commission standards but not their meanings or intents. For example, the *AMH* included standard chapters that were specific to physical rehabilitation and radiation oncology departments.

A survey consisted of surveyors arriving at the hospital with notice, spending lots of time in conversations with administration and subsequently burying themselves in paperwork. At hospitals, procedure manuals were removed from shelves and dusted off, and cover sheets were signed and readied for review. The "best" medical records were hand-picked and ready for the types of care that surveyors were most likely to inspect. If the surveyors traveled to your unit, it was more in the format of a tour and perhaps to engage in minimal conversation in an effort to impress upon staff members that they really did matter when it came to patient care.

For those of us who worked in the hospitals during this era, a Joint Commission survey was considered more of a bother than useful to improving care. Deficiencies we were hoping would be exposed were not discovered or were discussed behind closed doors. The medical staff interview consisted of an extravagant lunch and discussions that generally centered on the attendee's most recent golf game. Even if a hospital didn't meet Joint Commission standards, it could continue to attract business, treat patients, and receive payment in full for its services.

But then things began to change. Between 1987 and 1994, The Joint Commission continued to survey healthcare organizations by reviewing documentation, with an emphasis on retrospective assessment. Behind the scenes, however, The Joint Commission had embraced ideas based on total quality management put forth by W. Edwards Deming, and the concept of quality improvement. The accreditor started to rewrite its standards along those lines and called this process its "Agenda for Change."

Change in approach

In 1994, The Joint Commission unveiled its Agenda for Change and overhauled the *AMH*, renamed it the *Comprehensive Accreditation Manual for Hospitals (CAMH)*, and did away with the department-specific standards. The new standards were cross-functional and affected every department and staff member within an organization. The Agenda for Change placed a new emphasis on actual outcomes and results, rather than relying solely on measures of structure or process.

It also placed new demands on hospital staff members. Before the changes, departments had to concern themselves with only one section of the *AMH*. For example, nuclear medicine departments worried only about nuclear medicine standards, and dietitians focused only on dietetic standards. To meet the *CAMH*'s new cross-disciplinary standards, departments had to become familiar with the requirements of the Human Resources chapter, Infection Control chapter, Performance Improvement chapter, and so forth as processes affecting their departments were now dispersed throughout the manual.

Unfortunately, the mindset of some line managers has not transitioned from the "departmental think" of the early '90s into the cross-functional approach required today. For example, the Medication Management chapter is not applicable to only the pharmacy. Medication management standards apply to any location where medications are stored or administered.

> **Key Concept**
>
>
>
> Because the standards are applicable to many departments, consider asking a nonpharmacist to lead the Medication Management chapter team, and staff the team with a pharmacist and representatives from other applicable departments, such as interventional radiology, materials management, operating room, and of course, nursing.

Hospitals started to be surveyed on actual performance as well as on the quality of their plans or policies and how well different departments and disciplines work together to improve performance.

But the Agenda for Change didn't go far enough. The 1994 overhaul allowed hospitals to "gear up" for surveys by spending the year prior to (or in some cases, a couple of weeks before) the scheduled survey getting policies and procedures in shape and even painting and cleaning floors to create a good impression for surveyors. This system didn't seem the best way to measure what was really occurring in patient care.

The Joint Commission especially felt the pressure to examine its standards and survey process after the 1999 release of the Office of Inspector General report, "The External Review of Hospital Quality: The Role of Accreditation," which questioned the method of oversight of the accreditation process, and the Institute of Medicine (IOM) report, "To Err Is Human: Building a Safer Health System," which sounded a national alarm on the prevalence of medical errors in the United States.

The IOM report revealed that as many as 98,000 patients per year die from medical errors, making medical errors the eighth leading cause of death in the United States. The report called for a 50% reduction in medical errors in the following five years and recommended that The Joint Commission focus greater attention on safety.

When these reports were published, the public lost its confidence in The Joint Commission and in healthcare institutions. Hospitals felt pressure from patients, and The Joint Commission felt it from patient safety groups, hospitals, and the media, which criticized the accreditation process for failing to make healthcare safer. To restore public confidence and improve the quality and safety of healthcare organizations across the United States, the accreditor announced in the fall of 2002 that it would make significant changes to the accreditation process.

An overview of Shared Visions–New Pathways®

On January 1, 2004, The Joint Commission took the Agenda for Change one step further and introduced a new initiative it called Shared Visions–New Pathways, now more simply and commonly referred to as "the new survey process." The initiative focused on patient safety and quality and encouraged physicians to participate in the survey process. It also introduced healthcare organizations to a new set of consolidated standards and rules and new Joint Commission lingo, such as elements of performance (EP); A, B, and C category types; the PPR; the priority focus process; measures of success (MOS); evidence of standards compliance (ESC); clarification; and the centerpiece of the survey process, the tracer methodology.

In addition to consolidating standards, The Joint Commission changed how it scored the standards and required hospitals to complete a PPR—a lengthy, mid-cycle self-assessment tool to promote continuous standards compliance.

The survey process changed as well. During the Agenda for Change era, a Joint Commission survey involved 25% documentation review and 75% interaction with all levels of the staff in the hospital. The survey process today involves 10% documentation review and 90% interaction with staff members and patients at the "point of care" or at each patient care unit. Surveyors are on patient care units for a majority of the survey, asking for patient charts and then "tracing," or visiting, the same departments or services where the patients received treatment.

Chapter 1

Surveyors observe direct care, the medication process, and the care planning process; interview individual patients or families; review additional medical records; interview staff members about performance measurement; inquire about staff members' daily roles and responsibilities; and evaluate staff training and orientation. Surveyors also review policies and procedures as needed to clarify organizational expectations. Through their tracer activities, surveyors are able to assess a facility's compliance with standards and National Patient Safety Goals (NPSG).

Initially, hospital personnel were leery of the tracer methodology and were concerned that personnel would be unjustly subjected to questions that were outside their scope of practice. This did not hold true. In fact, just the opposite occurred. Based on our clients' feedback, personnel involved in tracer activities were excited that finally, individuals caring for the patients were included in the survey and that concurrent patient care was evaluated in place of retrospective chart review.

The Joint Commission expects an organization to be continuously ready for a survey. This is interpreted as meaning 100% compliance with all of The Joint Commission's standards, 100% of the time. In effect, if a surveyor unexpectedly shows up at your facility's door tomorrow, The Joint Commission expects that the organization will have all policies and procedures implemented and that staff members can answer questions a surveyor poses to them. In 2006, the survey process changed to an unannounced format to operationalize the expectation of continuous readiness.

January 2008: New president of The Joint Commission

Mark R. Chassin, MD, MPP, MPH, began his appointment as The Joint Commission's president on January 1, 2008.

During presentations in his first year with The Joint Commission, Chassin highlighted the initiation of Six Sigma improvement efforts within the internal operations of The Joint Commission. A major focus was on customer service, having listened to the feedback of the customers engaged in accreditation activities and their less than complimentary comments about some of The Joint Commission's processes, particularly surveyor variation regarding standards interpretation.

It is Chassin's belief that a "near miss" holds much value to institutions and is often not given the attention that is needed to avoid a more serious event. Near misses should be considered a wakeup call, an alert that the process is not consistently being carried out and should be promptly evaluated.

Joint Commission Makes Changes in Culture, Performance in 2009

The Joint Commission has made significant steps to improve its performance and culture in 2009, the organization announced during its recent Executive Briefings in New York.

Ann Scott Blouin, PhD, RN, executive vice president of accreditation and certification operations, discussed at length major changes the healthcare accrediting body has taken in recent months to improve the way it works with hospitals, as well as its own internal processes. Among those improvements:

- **Refocusing surveyors:** Blouin told the audience that The Joint Commission has refocused its 500 hospital surveyors to balance their roles as both evaluators and educators/coaches/mentors. According to Blouin, this was received as an invigorating change by 95% of the surveyors.

- **Adaptation:** The Joint Commission is using Lean, Six Sigma, and "change acceleration" to change its own culture. According to Blouin, there is a new focus on customer service and simplification of processes. The Joint Commission has also changed its tactics on criticality; now, only direct-impact RFIs affect accreditation decisions.

- **Post-survey reports:** The Joint Commission has promised to improve the time frame in which hospitals receive their post-survey reports. A recent study within the organization found that, on average, hospitals were receiving their reports 16.4 days after survey, with massive fluctuations in that time frame—despite a requirement that hospitals receive their report within 10 days of their survey (not a 10-day average). A new process has been developed to reduce the time to develop the report from 38 hours to 4.4 hours and the average time frame to receive the report to 5.4 days.

- **PPR:** The Joint Commission is examining changes and enhancements to the PPR based on feedback from the field that the dates of submission are not working.

And, as we discussed earlier this year, there are no more automatic thresholds—there is "no magic tipping point," says Blouin. The Joint Commission has also made a concerted effort to reduce costs.

Chapter 1

Unannounced survey process

The last group of hospitals that underwent the announced survey process in 2005 experienced their first unannounced survey in 2008, following the introduction of unannounced surveys for organizations due for survey in 2006. Organizations no longer know months in advance when surveyors will conduct their on-site visit for regular accreditation surveys.

All organizations are surveyed under the unannounced survey process with the following exceptions provided in the March 2009 edition of *Perspectives,* The Joint Commission's monthly publication (in which case surveys are announced):

Ambulatory care program

- All office-based surgical practices
- An organization that either provides nondeemed ambulatory surgery or telehealth, or is a sleep center

Behavioral health care program

- All methadone programs, if not part of a hospital
- All in-home behavioral health, case management, or Assertive Community Treatment programs, if not part of a hospital
- All freestanding organizations with 10 or fewer staff members or a total average daily census (ADC) of less than 100
- All community-based, freestanding programs

Home care program

- Small, nondeemed health and hospice organizations, if not part of a hospital

Medicare/Medicaid certification-based

- Long-term care program
- All one-day freestanding Medicare/Medicaid certification-based long-term care surveys, if not part of a hospital

- DCS certification programs
- All recertification reviews for lung volume reduction surgery and VAD

The Joint Commission considers the following to be the value of unannounced surveys:

- Greater focus on the changes that The Joint Commission makes throughout the year
- An end to "preparing to be surveyed" and a beginning to "preparing to embed the standards"
- Implementation of ongoing mock tracer activity to maintain continuous readiness

Can an unannounced survey be predicted?

Not at all. When unannounced surveys began in 2006, hospitals were told they would be surveyed anytime in the calendar year in which they were due for their triennial survey. However, this also has changed. As announced in the April 2008 issue of *Perspectives,* beginning as early as July 1, 2008, the survey window for hospitals could be as short as 18 months or as long as 39 months.

Field Experience

Undo energy is being spent to try to second-guess survey dates. The listservs are full of "creative research" highlighting ways you might be able to predict your survey date. In 2009, an organization was studying the time survey agendas posted on the Joint Commission Connect extranet and hypothesized that a survey would occur within two months of the posting. The question is: so what? What can we improve or correct within two months? Do we really want to revert to the game-playing of the early '90s? We would be far better off if we used our time to conduct tracers and continue to work our action plans for long-term fixes that improve standards compliance.

According to The Joint Commission, the timing of surveys is to be based on preestablished criteria generated from priority-focused process data and other data sources. In situations where the data suggest that patient safety and quality are potentially at risk, an organization will be scheduled for an earlier survey. The methods for calculating survey intervals are known by The Joint Commission and are not fully disclosed to accredited organizations. Read on and learn how the strategic surveillance system score was thought to have an impact on your next survey.

Strategic surveillance system

In July 2007, access to a Strategic Surveillance System (S3) score on the redesigned Joint Commission Connect extranet was initiated for the hospital accreditation program. This score is generated from a data management tool that operates as a dashboard, providing reports of comparative measures using data from:

- Past survey findings
- Core measures
- Complaints and non-self-reported sentinel events
- An organization's electronic application (e-App)
- Medicare Provider and Analysis Review (MedPAR)

At The Joint Commission's Executive Briefings held September 25, 2009, attendees were informed that scores from the Hospital Consumer Assessment of Healthcare Providers and Systems were added to the data used to formulate each hospital's S3 score. The Joint Commission also notified attendees that it was discussing the removal of MedPAR data but that no decision had been reached at that time.

Updated reports are posted quarterly on approximately the first of the month in April, July, and October. The S3 reports are only for use by hospitals via the secure, password-protected extranet site and are not available to the public.

Even though the S3 score has been available for some time, it is not unusual for a hospital's leadership team to be unaware of its organization's score. Not only does the report provide your facility's individual score, but it also lists your state scores and the national scores as well as comparison scores from the following groups:

- Top 10% of hospitals
- Top 25% of hospitals
- Thomson 100 Top Hospitals

- *U.S. News & World Report*'s America's Best Hospitals

- Magnet hospitals

- Hospitals undergoing for-cause surveys

- Hospitals receiving conditional accreditation

- Hospitals receiving preliminary denial of accreditation (PDA)

As the accreditation specialist, share the S3 score with your readiness teams, the performance improvement committee, the medical executive committee, and hospital leaders, including the board.

If we expect the leaders to be involved in promoting continuous standards compliance, measurement data such as the S3 score may be the impetus to push them into action or to keep the pressure on to maintain the best score possible. The S3 score is one situation where the lower the score, the better.

One of the reports available to organizations displays the percentage of the types of data used to calculate the S3 score. Unfortunately, data such as MedPAR results have such lag times that the information is considered outdated before it hits the S3 score. It is difficult to drill down into data which physicians and other staff members consider to be off the radar screen. It would take several years for implemented interventions to show an improvement. (Hence, this is a very good reason you should remove MedPAR results from the calculation of the S3 score.) In addition, it appears that hospitals with very high S3 scores have not been surveyed any earlier than those with lower scores.

Standards improvement initiative

In October 2006, The Joint Commission launched the Standards Improvement Initiative (SII) aimed at:

- Clarifying standards language

- Ensuring that standards are program-specific

- Deleting redundant and nonessential standards

- Consolidating standards

In August 2008, revised standards with scoring information were posted to The Joint Commission's Web site.

As a result of Phase I of the SII, the 2009 *CAMH* was published with five new chapters—Record of Care, Life Safety, Waived Testing, Transplant Services, and Emergency Management—for a total of 16 chapters. Type B EPs were eliminated, and we were introduced to new icons as highlighted in the following box:

> "Circle D": Required documentation, which may be in the form of a document or the act of documentation
>
> "Triangle 2": Indicates situational decisional rules (those listed in the ACC chapter of the standards manual that apply to conditional and predenial of accreditation)
>
> "Triangle 3": Indicates direct impact on patient safety and quality of care
>
> "Triangle 4": Indicates indirect impact on patient safety and quality of care (added in October 2009)
>
> "Circle M": Indicates an MOS is required if this EP was found to be noncompliant during the PPR or actual survey

In addition, a decimal system of standards numbering that leaves the reader confused as to how to locate a standard they knew well from the 2008 manual. The numbering system may help The Joint Commission, but it has caused confusion and persistent searching for the reader, also known as the customer.

EPs, standards, and scoring guidelines

In 2004, the fact that The Joint Commission initiated scoring based on an aggregation of an organization's compliance with all EPs caused some concern to hospitals undergoing survey. After all, Shared Visions–New Pathways was just as new to the surveyors as it was to organizations, and they feared the surveyors would overinterpret the EPs and put the hospital in accreditation jeopardy.

Even though we talk about standards being compliant or noncompliant, it is important to remember that scoring takes place at the EP level. As a result of the SSI, the EPs increased from approximately 1,200 to 1,700 in the hospital accreditation manual.

Category A EPs

These EPs are scored according to the presence (2 points) or absence (0 points) of the requirements (e.g., a policy, guidelines, etc.). An easy way to remember this category is "Either you have it, or you don't." There isn't any wiggle room.

Category C EPs

These EPs address issues that can be quantified or counted.

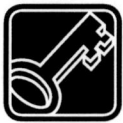

Key Concept

During the survey, category C EPs are scored based on the number of occurrences of noncompliance. No occurrences or even one occurrence is scored as compliant and is given two points. Two occurrences will yield a score of 1, which is partial compliance, and three or more occurrences equal noncompliance scored as a 0. Another way to remember this is "Three strikes and you're out."

Category C EPs are frequency-based during your survey but are rate-based when conducting an internal PPR. Ninety percent or greater compliance is considered full compliance, 80%–89% is partial compliance, and 79% or lower is scored as noncompliant. Remember: frequency-based during the survey, rate-based during PPR.

Scoring the standard

As I stated earlier, the EPs are actually where the initial scoring occurs. Anytime a single EP is scored as noncompliant, the standard is deemed noncompliant. The number of EPs is immaterial. It takes only one.

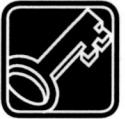

Key Concept

Not all hospital leaders have grasped this concept. If a noncompliant EP is identified and, if for some reason the leaders do not push for compliance, they need to be aware of the vulnerability that exists during a survey. The single noncompliant EP could lose the entire standard and increase the RFI count.

Based on the EP scores, a standard is scored as either compliant or noncompliant. At the conclusion of the survey, standards determined to be noncompliant are tagged as such and an RFI is generated.

Beginning in 2009, standards could no longer be scored as partially compliant as supplemental findings were discontinued. A standard that is not fully compliant will be considered a finding in which an RFI will be issued.

The introduction of criticality

The following four levels of criticality were introduced in 2009 as a method for focusing on EPs that have a greater impact on patient care and safety:

- Immediate Threat to Health and Safety
- Situational Decision Rules
- Direct Impact Requirements
- Indirect Impact Requirements

If you are experienced with CMS surveys, the term *immediate jeopardy* should be familiar. The concepts here are similar to Immediate Threat to Health and Safety as there is not a specific listing of causes that can result in this finding, but the following examples were listed in the 2009 *CAMH:*

- Inoperable fire alarm
- Adult-strength medications on pediatric crash cart
- Lack of master alarms for medical gas systems
- Patients with known antibodies receiving transfusions without the units being typed for the corresponding antigen

The seriousness of this determination yields an expedited decision of PDA. A follow-up survey is required to clear the PDA decision. Even after the immediate threat has been corrected, the organization receives conditional accreditation until a follow-up survey is performed within four to six months.

The next level of criticality, Situational Decision Rules, is based on specific situations identified during the survey. The following examples were provided in the 2009 *CAMH*:

- A facility without a license

- An individual without a license when a license is required

- Failure to implement *Life Safety Code® (LSC)* corrective actions

EPs that are subject to this level of criticality are labeled with a black triangle that has a "2" in it. Depending on the finding, a decision of either PDA or conditional accreditation could be rendered. During this year, *Perspectives* addressed this topic as it tends to be overwhelming to hospitals. In the *CAMH*, the tab labeled "ACC" provides a lengthy listing of accreditation decisions known as "Rules" that provide the reader with a more thorough explanation that is beyond the scope of this publication.

New Accreditation Decision

What Will This Mean for Your Facility?
The Joint Commission has announced it will adopt a new accreditation decision for 2010. This decision, "Medicare Condition-Level Deficiency Follow-Up Survey," is intended when surveyors assess a facility with one or more condition-level deficiencies out of compliance.

These condition-level deficiencies refer specifically to the CMS *CoP*s. This new accreditation decision is based in part on the Joint Commission's application for hospital deeming authority through CMS.

According to The Joint Commission, if and when an organization has received this decision following a survey, the organization must address the identified deficient *CoP*s. After this, a follow-up survey will be conducted on-site. The Joint Commission has specifically stated that this accreditation decision is not to be confused with conditional accreditation decisions.

"I'm sure this is the result of continuing dialogue between The Joint Commission and CMS regarding the Joint Commission's pending deeming application decision," says **Joe Cappiello,** chair of Cappiello & Associates in Elmhurst, IL. "What CMS probably said was, 'If you have a condition out, it has to be fixed right away, and you'll have to go back in there and validate that it was fixed.'" This initial announcement did not address what scenarios will cause this type of accreditation decision.

New Accreditation Decision (Cont.)

What Will Trigger a Visit?

A number of events could trigger a post-survey on-site visit, says Cappiello. Here are a few possible examples:

- **Post-survey random unannounced survey:** "This is the 5% random sample pool that everyone is put in," says Cappiello. "If you require submission of an MOS, you are out of the pool until your MOS is submitted."

- **Post-submission of clarifying data:** "If the initial decision was conditional or [a] preliminary denial of accreditation," says Cappiello, "[an] on-site clarification validation survey [CVS] will be scheduled if [the] clarification changed the accreditation decision."

Other hypothetical causes for this survey include:

- Conditional decision follow-up survey
- ESC survey
- MOS survey
- Sentinel event follow-up survey
- *CoP* follow-up survey

"With the exception of the *CoP* follow-up survey, these are just [a] part of the previously published accreditation process," says Cappiello. As another example, say your hospital does not exceed the bandwidth but receives a few RFIs. If you have a *CoP* out, that will require a follow-up visit.

What The Joint Commission didn't reveal, says Cappiello, was the time frame. Historically, CMS requires correction and verification by on-site follow-up within 90 days. "I would imagine that CMS will require The Joint Commission to follow that timeline," says Cappiello.

As yet another example, say you've exceeded your bandwidth, you have gone to conditional accreditation, and you have a *CoP* out. This means you'll get a follow-up conditional survey by The Joint Commission following your acceptable submission of ESC and you'll have a follow-up by The Joint Commission based on the *CoP*s.

> **New Accreditation Decision (Cont.)**
>
> "We don't know if those two are combined," says Cappiello. "Would they do them at the same time? Come back and take a look at direct impact standards and *CoP*s in the same visit? But what if the timelines are not compatible? I would hope that if the timelines match, The Joint Commission would combine the two into a single visit." If, however, the timelines turn out to be incompatible, this could result in two visits—both of which the hospital pays for.
>
> This may also have an effect on the size of the team sent for the follow-up survey. A follow-up survey frequently comprises one surveyor for one day. If a number of standards and a number of *CoP*s are out, this may result in a larger review team. "I would think that The Joint Commission would review the timeline and the size/composition of the survey team on an individual basis," says Cappiello. Also unclear at this point are the number of post-survey processes.
>
> "Let's say the report has been issued and the decision has been rendered," says Cappiello. "How soon after the organization receives the report is this new condition-level deficiency follow-up done? Do they need to submit to The Joint Commission just like they do to [CMS] a plan of correction? What are they requiring to be submitted prior to the follow-up, and how far out will that be scheduled?"
>
> Source: **Briefings on The Joint Commission,** September 2009.

The third criticality level, Direct Impact Requirements, is the icon that we tend to watch for more often. EPs labeled with a white triangle with a "3" inside are based on implementation of care processes, and if noncompliance exits there are few or no protective defenses to prevent an impact on patient quality and safety. It is the number of noncompliant standards determined by noncompliant direct impact EPs that may cause the surveyors to look for patterns or trends in their findings.

The concept of program-specific bands for determining screening thresholds for more intense evaluation of findings for the number of noncompliant direct impact standards was introduced with surveys beginning in 2009. Determining your organization's screening threshold is a two-step process. First, you must calculate the number of surveyor days, by simply adding the number of surveyors and the number of days they were on-site for your most recent survey or as described in your survey agenda posted on the Joint Commission's Connect extranet.

For example, say that three surveyors were on-site for three days, plus another surveyor was there for two days: 3 * 3 = 9 + 2 = 11. For a hospital with 11 surveyor days, the organization is placed in Band 4 based on Table 1 found in the "HB" section of the *CAMH* updated in June 2009.

In Table 2, Band 4 depicts 11 noncompliant direct impact standards as the screening level for a review by the central office of The Joint Commission.

Do the bands still exist?

At the same September Executive Briefings presentation mentioned earlier in this chapter, additional information was provided to the audience regarding direct impact bands. Here is a summary of the topic:

There are no "magic numbers" that result in adverse action, even though the surveyor days/bands have been published. According to all three speakers at the presentation, never have specific numbers rendered an organization immediately into adverse action. That concept (according to all three speakers) has been a misconception by the industry since the publication of the bands. The issue with the number of RFIs apparently is to evaluate for trends or for significance of the RFIs. Adverse action should occur only if there was a negative trend or pattern with the types of standards scored as noncompliant. For example, if several RFIs trended in life safety and leadership (because leadership wasn't performing its oversight function), adverse action may occur. Each report would be reviewed individually. A member of the Joint Commission staff was asked this question: "If a small hospital had 20 direct impact RFIs and none of them were related and did not roll up into a trend of any kind, would there be no adverse action?" The spokesperson replied, "No. There would not." The next question: "How, then, in this scenario, would the hospital's accreditation status read?" The reply: "Simply, accredited with RFIs."

With this new information, the organization should perhaps consider that its number of direct impact RFIs would be a trigger for the surveyors to look more carefully at the type and patterns of the RFIs. Stay tuned for more clarification from The Joint Commission.

Direct impact noncompliant standards are to be corrected within 45 days following survey. This was a change effective in 2009 to have different time frames for achieving standards compliance.

The final criticality level is Indirect Impact Requirements. New information provided on page 12 of *Perspectives* announces that a symbol for the indirect impact findings is a triangle with a 4 inside. EPs considered to be indirect have to do with planning and evaluation of care processes. If noncompliance is not resolved, there is still a risk to the patient's quality and safety, but initially, not at the level of the direct impact EPs.

If no direct impact EPs are found to be noncompliant (partials included), noncompliant indirect EPs would result in a noncompliant indirect standard. The organization will have up to 60 days to correct this finding following survey.

And the changes continued

Just a little more than three months after hospitals received their 2009 edition of *CAMH,* The Joint Commission released a document on its Web site titled "New & Revised 2009 Accreditation Requirements in Response to CMS Deeming Application." Hospitals were stunned: 46 pages of approximately 165 EPs in addition to the previous changes in the 2009 standards scoring; numbering; more chapters; NPSGs; and now this. To make things worse, a July 1, 2009, implementation was expected.

Accreditation specialists scrambled to meet these new requirements. Valuable resources were being expended when, on March 26, 2009, yet another revision was posted! This document decreased the EP changes to 87 and eliminated some of the EPs that hospitals had already implemented. Sound familiar? It should. And one of the most damaging fallouts to the accreditation specialists was that staff members, including physicians, were beginning to question the credibility of the messenger and The Joint Commission.

Damage control began as well as the review of the March 26 revisions. To ensure that you are on target, Chapter 2 will focus on these changes and offer suggestions for compliance. Even though hospitals received the updates in June, some seem to have slipped by without adequate attention; hence, the reason for Chapter 2.

The Survey Process

The Joint Commission has not announced any changes to the actual on-site survey process for 2010. You can find a full description of the components of a survey in The Joint Commission's *Survey Activity Guide,* last published in January 2009 and available on the Joint Commission Connect extranet. We will discuss additional recommendations for preparing and managing survey readiness in Chapter 7 of this book.

Individual tracers

If you were to ask hospital staff members about the most significant change in the survey process in recent years, they would likely respond that it is the implementation of tracers. Subsequent to their introduction in 2004, tracers make up most survey activities; the actual number depends on the length of your organization's survey.

Patients are selected for tracers from the census provided each morning to the surveyors. An "ideal" patient is one who has been in the hospital several days but not much longer than seven days; otherwise, the medical record is too extensive and time-consuming for performing a thorough tracer. Generally, patients with diagnoses from the organization's clinical service groups will be selected.

Upon arrival to the patient care unit, the surveyor will ask to meet with the caregiver assigned to the patient. At this point, the surveyor begins the assessment process. As the caregiver prepares to meet with the surveyor, the process of handoff communication will be closely observed.

The tracer activity begins at the point that the patient entered your organization. If the tracer is being conducted in the medical unit, it is possible that the patient was admitted via the emergency department, may have been a patient in the intensive care unit, and may have undergone diagnostic testing with a subsequent admission. Surveyors expect that caregivers can locate information from all aspects of the medical record. Otherwise, continuity of care is broken and nonexistent.

Examples of dos and don'ts to follow

Do:

Preselect a location for conducting tracers in each patient care unit. Staff members do not need the added stress of juggling records while surveyors are becoming agitated as they wait for a review site to be selected. If your medical record is electronic, be sure to plan for a computer to be available in the selected review location.

Once you've been notified that the surveyors have arrived to conduct your unannounced survey, ensure that the selected location is clear of debris and that adequate seating exists for the surveyor, the caregiver, the surveyor escort, and perhaps one additional person. Test the computer to be used for tracers to ensure that it is functional. Collect all components of the hardcopy medical record, including those that might be stored separately from the primary medical record, such as medication administration records, care plans, and so forth.

Remind the patient caregiver of the patient selected for the tracer to hand off to another caregiver. Surveyors tend to watch this practice very carefully.

Don't:

Attempt to answer for staff members participating in the tracer or try to provide prompts when answers are not readily articulated. The tracer is an activity between the surveyor and the assigned caregiver. Managers should not be involved, as this could spur an invitation to exit the activity.

Expound too much on answers. Doing so will often reveal information that exposes deficiencies in care that were outside the scope of the surveyor's question.

Be defensive. Defensiveness has no place in tracer activity; if a deficiency in documentation is identified and it is from a previous unit or caregiver, accept the fact of the deficiency and answer questions as asked. Comments such as "Oh, this field should have contained the pain assessment" may seem minor, but in our state of nervousness, we might let such a comment slip. The solution is to practice the survey process with another department manager to ensure that your conduct remains appropriate.

Attempt to answer a question by assuming what the documentation was intended to mean; let the record speak for itself.

Using the preceding example, if medical unit staff members are unable to locate the pain assessment performed in the emergency department, for instance, it becomes obvious to the surveyor that the receiving unit does not utilize this information and that caregivers may be practicing within their own silo of care.

> **Success Story**
>
>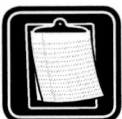
>
> The transition to electronic records is not an easy conversion, and it becomes particularly troublesome during a tracer when staff members are under the gun to locate specific information. One organization developed a road map for nursing staff members who were still struggling with computer documentation. Snapshots of key screens and highlighted fields were printed in small tiles with step-by-step instructions detailing how to open the screens. Based on this information, the emergency department triage form and the pain assessment field were identified. The road maps were laminated and were used in daily work to increase their computer expertise.
>
> As the surveyor questions the caregiver, notes will be taken about the other units in which the patient received care. Expect to travel to those units next. This will continue until the surveyor has exhausted the patient care locations or time has lapsed for the selected patient tracer.

In addition to individual patient tracers, system tracers were introduced in 2004, others were added in 2006, and program-specific tracers were added in 2008. System tracers include the following:

Medication management (MM)

This session is designed to explore the organization's MM practices and to identify any potential risks. The specific medication processes that surveyors will look at include medication storage, ordering, transcribing, administration, and monitoring. Following a group discussion, it is likely that a patient receiving either complex medications or a medication listed on the organization's list of high-alert medications will be selected for a review of medication practices. This may begin either in the pharmacy or on the patient care unit and will involve tracing the medications from the time of order through to administration.

> **Key Concept**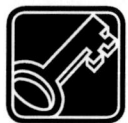
>
> A thorough medication tracer may be based on actual findings identified before this system tracer. A medication tracer typically begins with questions regarding the licensed independent practitioner's order. Be prepared to articulate whether standing orders, protocols, and preprinted order sets are allowed. The process of the order being received by the pharmacy, pharmacist review, transfer to a medication administration record, and administration is game for discussion. If the appropriate parties are not initially included in the tracer, it is acceptable to summons them. However, if staff members in attendance should know the listed processes but do not, a red flag will go up and digging will begin into policies and procedures.

Infection control (IC)

Discussions of the hospital's IC program will usually begin with a review of the annual risk analysis, prioritization of risks, strategies for reducing risks, and measurements of progress. Surveillance data should be readily available for this discussion. Surveyors may subsequently request the name of a patient currently in isolation and conduct a review of the record within the patient care unit. In the *Survey Activity Guide,* IC data are listed as the document to have ready for the surveyor's review. Be prepared with a list of patients currently in isolation, the most current risk analysis, the prioritized strategies, and recent measurement data of the strategies.

Data use

The participants in this session should be well prepared to discuss data collection, data analysis, selection of appropriate interventions, and subsequent measurement to assess effectiveness. Surveyors generally focus on data used to improve the safety and quality of care, such as medication errors, patient falls, use of restraints and seclusion, organ procurement conversion rate, and perhaps any of the other topics listed in PI.01.01.01.

> **Field Experience**
>
> Accreditation specialists report variation from the description of this system tracer in the *Survey Activity Guide.* It seems that some surveyors bring forth findings from individual tracers and ask for data to prove or disprove those findings. Others have indicated that surveyors do most of the talking and address only the data provided in the document review session on the first day of the survey. Regardless of these reports, be prepared in accordance to the preceding description.

Emergency management (EM)

The EM tracer was established in 2006 for hospitals with more than 200 licensed beds, and in 2008, it was expanded to include all hospitals, regardless of size. This tracer was added in the aftermath of a review of the challenges hospitals faced during events such as the Gulf Coast hurricanes, including Katrina; the floods in Houston; and other catastrophic events in which response capabilities were quickly reduced to the point of evacuation.

During this tracer, surveyors will review and assess your hazard vulnerability analysis; your organization's role in relation to the community's EM planning; your preparations relative to the key response functions (communications, resources and assets, safety and security, staff, utility systems, patient care); practical implementation of the "all hazards" incident command structure (including linkages with the community); your organization's capabilities during long-term events with no support from the community; and improvements made in response to opportunities identified during EM exercises.

In some instances, surveyors have been known to travel to specific patient care unit(s) and pose an emergency scenario (nominally based on your hazard vulnerability analysis), and then interview staff members within the unit on their role in EM. Consider adding a brief EM tracer to environmental rounds as a method to practice spontaneous questioning to staff members who may not be expecting to participate in EM survey activities.

> **Key Concept**
>
> And just as we thought we were over the need to pull closed records for Joint Commission surveys, a change in the on-site survey process was published in the October 2009 issue of *Perspectives*. Effective immediately, for general acute care hospitals (not for specialty hospitals), at least 10% of the ADC, but not fewer than 30 records, are to be reviewed during the survey. Included is a qualifier for small general hospitals, but a definition of what is considered small was not provided. The example was a hospital with an ADC of 20 and that 20 records reviewed might be adequate if the surveyors could assess compliance. It seems a clearer definition is warranted.

Typically, record review has occurred during individual and system tracers, but the numbers of reviews depended on the length of the survey and number of surveyors. Agendas are packed with multiple activities now, so the first question is how the additional record review will occur. And think about this: If you have recently changed a process to comply with a standard, retrospective chart review might include those who received care prior to the change. Yikes, the olden days have returned with the influence from CMS. The good news is that the Joint Commission survey process will certainly prepare you for the dreaded CMS arrival because it appears that the two organizations' survey processes are becoming increasingly similar.

What is the possible effect on your organization? For a medium-size hospital with an ADC of 130, 10% would be 13 records. An additional 17 records will need to be included in the review process to reach 30 records. Historically, your on-site survey has been scheduled for three days with three surveyors for clinical activities, not counting the life safety surveyor. Based on the typical three-day agenda, there are 19 opportunities for chart reviews during tracers. An additional 11 records, either open or closed, would need to be requested for review.

Sentinel events

We should all know that a sentinel event is any unexpected death or serious physical or psychological injury (e.g., loss of limb or function) to a patient. The Joint Commission initiated this term and the investigation of such events in 1998.

An organization is not required to report a sentinel event to The Joint Commission, but it is required to conduct a thorough and credible root-cause analysis that includes an extensive action plan to reduce the risks of such an event occurring again. Joint Commission surveyors are instructed not to inquire about the occurrence of sentinel events, but they may ask staff members about methods for reporting such events and the subsequent investigation process. Should The Joint Commission become aware of a sentinel event, its inquiry will be directed to the contact people listed on your facility's e-App; alternatively, depending on the circumstances, a for-cause survey could be triggered. Consult your standards manual for more information on this topic.

The Joint Commission periodically releases Sentinel Event Alerts. One of the most recent such alerts is Leadership Committed to Safety, which The Joint Commission posted on its Web site on August 27, 2009, and revised on September 8, 2009. These alerts include occurrence data, strategies for risk reduction, and recommendations for preventing the event. As a component of accreditation, organizations are no longer required to assess the application of the recommendations and implement those that are appropriate. The question to you as an accreditation specialist and promoter of patient safety is why you would not want to utilize this valuable information already packaged for your review. It is recommended that each Sentinel Event Alert be assessed for implementation of recommendations as applicable to your hospital's services and population. Also consider using the analysis of the alert and application to your organization as your required 18-month proactive risk assessment, formerly known as a Failure Modes and Effects Analysis.

Electronic application

Hospitals have access to their e-App that is available on the Joint Commission Connect extranet. Your assigned Joint Commission account executive is able to assist you in updating the application and answering content questions. Surveyors also are able to access the application via their laptops.

It is imperative that your organization's e-App remains current. You must report any addition or deletion of a service to The Joint Commission within 30 days of the occurrence.

If you are questioning the necessity of reporting a change, contact your Joint Commission account executive for advice. Should you miss the 30-day deadline and the changes in service are adding significant patient volume, this could trigger an extension survey.

In addition, the application is utilized to plan the length of the on-site survey, the number of surveyors, and the specific qualifications of a surveyor should your facility include home care, behavioral health services, and so forth.

Your Survey Team

Generally, The Joint Commission sends a team comprising a physician, a nurse, and an administrator to survey a hospital, and one of these three people acts as the survey team leader. Surveys last for two to five days, depending on the number of beds in your hospital and the scope of your patient care activities.

For a hospital with fewer than 50 beds, for example, The Joint Commission typically sends a physician and nurse surveyor for two days. A survey at a facility with 500 to 750 beds would likely involve four surveyors and last at least four to five days. Beginning in 2008, all hospitals had an additional *LSC* surveyor for one day, and if the facility met specific square footage requirements, a second day was added.

The Joint Commission also may add more surveyors to a team if necessary. For example, if travel to a hospital's outlying ambulatory campuses is necessary, The Joint Commission might send an additional surveyor for those sites.

Also, The Joint Commission might assign additional surveyors to review specialty areas, such as home health, long-term care, and nursing home facilities affiliated with a hospital. Check your survey agenda once it is posted to the extranet for hospital-specific information.

TEST YOUR KNOWLEDGE

1. True or false: If your organization is accredited by The Joint Commission, you will be exempt from full surveys conducted by CMS.

Answer: False. The Joint Commission accreditation grants your organization "deemed status" to bill Medicare and Medicaid for services provided. CMS still provides oversight to all entities with deemed status. Validation surveys, follow-ups on complaints, and so forth may still be performed by CMS.

2. Which of the following is true regarding scoring of standards?
    A. Partial compliance will result in a supplemental finding
    B. Indirect impact requirements scored as noncompliant must be resolved within 45 days
    C. Immediate Threat to Health and Safety may result in either a preliminary denial of accreditation or conditional accreditation
    D. Conditional accreditation due to a situational decision rule must be corrected within 45 days

Answer: D. Evidence of standards compliance must be submitted to The Joint Commission within 45 days. A follow-up validation survey will also be conducted.

CHAPTER 2

Addressing the Changes in Standards for 2009

We mentioned in Chapter 1 that The Joint Commission was required to reapply to the Centers for Medicare & Medicaid Services (CMS) for deemed status. As a result, in January 2009, The Joint Commission posted new and revised standards to the Internet, with an expectation that the standards would be implemented by July 1, 2009. Readers immediately noted the increased references to *Conditions of Participation (CoP)* numbers as The Joint Commission revised its standards to incorporate *CoP*s that were not previously represented. Just two months later, on March 26, 2009, The Joint Commission reissued the January standards, reducing the number of total standards but keeping the same implementation date. As a result of discussions between The Joint Commission and CMS, fewer changes were needed.

Instructions with the second release indicated that the standards were an addendum to the current standards. Beginning on April 6 and through June 30, 2009, surveyors evaluated the new and revised standards, but if they identified any noncompliance they did not include their findings in their accreditation decision.

Even though the implementation date has long passed, it appears that some of the standards were either overlooked or interpreted incorrectly, as noncompliance is being seen when consulting assessments are conducted. Therefore, this chapter will illustrate which elements of performances (EP) may be falling through the cracks at your facility and, as appropriate, offer suggestions for compliance. Please refer to the *Comprehensive Accreditation Manual for Hospitals (CAMH)* for the complete wording of these EPs; I will only paraphrase them in this chapter.

Standard and Element of Performance	Intent
HR.01.04.01 EP 3	Staff members will be oriented to relevant hospital policies and procedures; this will be documented.

Documentation of this process is not occurring. Most organizations utilize a checklist to document the topics that are included in departmental orientation. Add an entry of "relevant policies and procedures." Do not overdo this, however; a listing of all the policies is not required.

Standard and Element of Performance	Intent
LD.04.01.05 EP 7	The services of anesthesia, nuclear medicine, and respiratory care are directed by a qualified physician.

This is not usually a problem in larger facilities, but for smaller hospitals it seems that respiratory care in particular may not be under the direction of a qualified physician. The standards do not define what constitutes as "qualified"; as such, the hospital should define what this means based on the complexity of the services provided.

Standard and Element of Performance	Intent
LS.01.01.01 EP 4	Documents generated from state or local fire control agencies are to be maintained by the hospital.

One would expect this to be a common practice, but in the past when management was asked to produce these documents, retrieval was not so easy. In some situations, the facility director had to contact the agencies for copies of previous inspections. Ensure that this is a component of your organization's life safety files and that these documents can be readily located, if requested.

Standard and Element of Performance	Intent
MM.01.01.03 EP 5	Abuses and losses of controlled substances are to be reported to the pharmacy director and, as determined by the organization, to the CEO. Laws and regulations are to be followed.

If you were asked to produce a policy or procedure related to management of controlled substances, could you rapidly locate the document? It sounds easy, but it seems that the keeper is generally the pharmacy director and others are not familiar with the process. Take a moment to talk with your pharmacy director and determine whether such a document exists. Ensure that it includes who must be notified of abuses and losses and which laws and regulations are applicable in your state.

Standard and Element of Performance	Intent
MM.05.01.07 EP 5	Licensed independent practitioners (LIP) order medications that are to be prepared and administered.

Remember the debate that ensued in late 2008 when CMS revised its *CoPs* and included a requirement similar to this EP? The Joint Commission later distributed a memo, and shortly afterward so did CMS, saying they were revising the requirement as they did not intend to prevent the delivery of emergency and necessary care. Subsequent clarification was to be published, but as of the time of this writing, nothing has been released. In your facility, an order could be defined as a protocol, standing order, preprinted orders, clinical pathways, or practice guidelines, just to name a few. This is a difficult topic, and we will discuss it further in Chapter 3.

Standard and Element of Performance	Intent
MS.01.01.01 EP 20	The requirements for a history and physical (H&P) are to be included in the medical staff bylaws.

The issue here is that this type of information has historically been described in the medical staff rules and regulations. There continues to be a debate as to whether the rules and regulations are an addendum to the medical staff bylaws or whether they are a separate document. This seems to be trivial and not worth debating. The more important focus should be on whether H&Ps are being completed within the defined time frames and contain the appropriate information. If the medical staff bylaws reference the rules and regulations as an addendum, which is most commonly included toward the end of the bylaws, consider it done!

Standard and Element of Performance	Intent
MS.03.01.01 EP 13	Off-campus patient care sites are to have a medical staff–approved policy for appraisal of emergencies, initial treatment, and referral.

Locate your hospital's policy regarding management of patient emergencies. If off-site locations have not been addressed, determine the most appropriate emergency response and add it to the existing policy. Consider the mix of staff members at the off-site locations whenever patients are present. Are they trained to initiate emergency care? If a crash cart is present in the facility, do you have LIPs who are trained in providing advanced cardiac life support on-site? What about pediatric patients? If this population is included in the scope of services, are pediatric medications and supplies available that are equal to those for adults?

Remember, it is perfectly acceptable to initiate CPR and to call 911. Be careful not to increase your organization's liability by having equipment and medications available without staff members who are trained to use and administer them. Also, this EP contains a key requirement: medical staff–written policies and procedures. If you have an existing policy, ensure that the medical director of emergency services or the medical executive committee has approved it, or that it has gone through some other method of medical staff approval.

Standard and Element of Performance	Intent
MS.06.01.03 EP 9	A full-time, part-time, or consulting radiologist supervises ionizing radiology services.

This is similar to the leadership standard previously discussed and may be more of a problem in smaller facilities. Note that a radiologist is required and that radiologists should not be confused with radiation safety officers who are typically radiation physicists.

Standard and Element of Performance	Intent
PC.02.01.01 EP 1 and EP 7	EP 1: LIPs provide orders prior to the delivery of care, treatment, and services. EP 7: The most recent patient order is utilized.

These two EPs are similar, so I am addressing both of them here. The patient care location at increased risk for noncompliance to these EPs is the emergency department. During periods of high census, verbal orders may have been provided but not documented. Or a physician may be occupied with a critical patient and an experienced nurse may initiate care outside the scope of nursing prior to obtaining an order. Some organizations continue to use outdated "preference cards" that describe medications and diagnostic tests that the physician desires for each patient. Preference cards are not orders. Because these tie in with the various order types previously listed in standard MM.05.01.07 EP 5, a more in-depth discussion of orders will appear in Chapter 3.

EP 7 becomes a problem when the anesthesia provider, the surgeon, and the medical doctor write medication orders. What a nightmare for the pharmacist who is reviewing multiple analgesic orders and attempting to determine which one is the most "current." One hospital solved this dilemma by delegating pain control to the anesthesia provider while the patient remained in the post-anesthesia care unit (PACU). Once the patient was transferred to the surgical unit, the surgeon's analgesic orders were followed.

An electronic medication administrative record (MAR) helps the nurse to determine which order is the most current. As medication orders expire, they are dropped from the MAR. If you are using a hard-copy MAR, ensure that the date of the order is recorded.

Standard and Element of Performance	Intent
PC.03.01.03 EP 18	Within 48 hours prior to surgery or a procedure requiring anesthesia, a preanesthesia evaluation is performed.

Within this standard, the old standby of EP 1 still remains. EP 1 requires a hospital to conduct a presedation or preanesthesia assessment, but a time frame is not included. The new EP is a carryover from CMS where its emphasis is on anesthesia and not sedation. The 48-hour time frame will be important if your facility has implemented preoperative anesthesia evaluations earlier than 48 hours prior to surgery. Some hospitals implemented earlier preop testing and anesthesia evaluations to enable outpatient billing separate from the diagnosis-related group. This new EP will prevent that type of reimbursement strategy.

Chapter 2

Standard and Element of Performance	Intent
PC.03.01.07 EP 7 and EP 8	EP 7: An individual qualified to administer anesthesia must conduct a post-anesthesia evaluation no later than 48 hours after surgery or a procedure requiring anesthesia. EP 8: The medical staff is to approve the policy requiring the 48-hour post-anesthesia evaluation.

Many hospitals have already implemented these EPs because they have been a CMS requirement for years. For hospitals that have focused on the Joint Commission standards and pretty much pushed the CMS *CoPs* back into the closet, implementing these EPs could be a challenge.

Notice that this EP does not specify inpatients versus outpatients, nor does it exclude the PACU anesthesia visit as fulfilling this requirement. The purpose of the evaluation is to determine whether the patient recovered from anesthesia without suffering any complications. Because the definition of anesthesia includes spinals and blocks, the time period for performing the evaluation for these two types of anesthesia would need to be greater than what could be assessed in the PACU. When the patient has recovered from general anesthesia, it would be acceptable to perform the post-evaluation in the PACU.

A simple way to track patients requiring a post-anesthesia assessment is to maintain a hard copy of the daily surgery schedule in the anesthesia department. Each morning, an anesthesia provider is assigned to perform inpatient post-anesthesia visits. Some hospitals have utilized the same anesthesia provider to perform preanesthesia assessments for hospitalized patients.

Before considering whether your organization complies with this EP, you should collect data as a component of medical record review. Consider including the results of this data collection in the practitioner profile for anesthesia providers.

Restraint and Seclusion

A few words about the restraint standards and EPs are in order, as this topic can be confusing. First, it was not clear that hospitals using the Joint Commission accreditation for deemed status were to replace the entire section of standards addressing restraints and seclusion in the 2009 *CAMH* with the standards released in March 2009. This was clarified in the May 2009 edition of *Perspectives*. Second, accreditation specialists around the country were trying to make sense of the new lingo, retrofit newly created standards into the complicated numbering system, and attempt to sort out what was minimally required. Client questions exploded and the answers were impossible to obtain. Third, the May 2009 issue of *Perspectives* did not address whether the Record of Care standards regarding data collection were still applicable.

The June 2009 issue of *Perspectives* finally announced that hospitals using The Joint Commission for deemed status purposes were to ignore RC.02.01.05 regarding documentation of restraint usage. Because The Joint Commission has only microscopically assessed the issue of restraints, hospitals are hesitant to revise their current policies and change their practices from the historically more restrictive Joint Commission standards to the more lenient standards. To assist in transitioning to a more simplified approach to restraint usage, I provide the following sample policy for your review and use.

Model Policy: Restraint and Seclusion

A. DEFINITIONS

Restraint is any manual method, physical or mechanical device, material, or equipment that immobilizes or reduces the ability of a patient to move his or her arms, legs, body, or head freely. (Refer to Attachment A for exceptions from and examples of restraint.)

Seclusion is the involuntary confinement of a patient alone in a room or an area from which he or she is physically prevented from leaving. (Refer to Attachment A for exclusions from and examples of seclusion.)

Chemical restraint is the use of a medication to restrict a patient's freedom of movement that is not a standard treatment for the patient's new or continuing medical or behavioral condition. It is this hospital's policy to only use medications that are a standard treatment for the patient's ongoing or newly emerging condition. Therefore, chemical restraint is not used in this institution.

Model Policy: Restraint and Seclusion (Cont.)

B. GENERAL PROVISIONS

Indications:

- Restraint or seclusion may be used when less restrictive means would not be effective to protect the physical safety of patients, a staff member, or others

- Seclusion may be used only for the management of violent or self-destructive behavior that jeopardizes the immediate safety of the patient, a staff member, or others

Initiation: Each episode of restraint or seclusion shall be initiated in one of the following circumstances:

- Upon the order of a licensed independent practitioner (LIP) who is responsible for the patient

- By a registered nurse if necessary to protect the patient, staff members, or others from harm, provided that an order is obtained from an LIP who is responsible for the patient as soon as possible after initiation

Notification of the attending physician: If the attending physician is not the person who ordered the restraint, he or she shall be notified that restraint was applied (e.g., through review of the restraint order) by the end of the calendar day following initiation of the restraint order. (Documentation of any kind by the attending physician, whether or not it addresses restraint, shall constitute sufficient evidence that the attending physician was notified of the restraint episode.)

PRN orders: PRN orders for restraint or seclusion shall not be used.

Exceptions: A standing or PRN order may be used for the following interventions:

- The patient requires the use of a Geri chair with the tray locked to be safe out of bed
- Bed side rails are used as restraint (refer to Attachment A)
- Interventions are used to protect the patient from repetitive self-mutilating behavior

Duration of restraint/orders:

- Orders for restraint or seclusion applied to manage violent or self-destructive behavior that jeopardizes the immediate safety of the patient, a staff member, or others shall

Model Policy: Restraint and Seclusion (Cont.)

- remain in effect until the patient's behavior or situation no longer requires the use of restraint or seclusion, but for no longer than:
    - Four hours for adults 18 years of age or older
    - Two hours for children and adolescents 9–17 years of age
    - One hour for children 8 years of age or younger

Renewal orders may be given for the preceding durations if the indications for restraint or seclusion persist. However, continuation of restraint or seclusion for longer than 24 hours shall be based on an in-person evaluation by a responsible LIP.

- Physician orders for restraint that is not used for management of violent or self-destructive behavior shall remain in effect until one of the following occurs:
    - The patient's behavior or situation no longer requires the use of restraint
    - The indications for discontinuation listed on the medical staff–approved protocol are met
    - The end of the calendar day following the date of the order when a medical staff–approved protocol is not used

Assessment and monitoring

Restraint/seclusion monitoring and assessments shall include at least the elements indicated on the current version of the approved nursing assessment forms and flowsheets.

- Management of violent or self-destructive behavior that jeopardizes the immediate safety of the patient, a staff member, or others:
    - **One-hour face-to-face assessment:** A responsible LIP, a registered nurse, or a physician assistant shall perform a face-to-face assessment of the patient's physical and psychological status within one hour of the initiation of restraint or seclusion. Registered nurses or physician assistants who perform such assessments shall be trained as specified in Section C.2 of this policy.
    - **Monitoring:** Restrained or secluded patients shall be subject to monitoring by individuals trained according to Sections C.2 and C.3 of this policy.

Model Policy: Restraint and Seclusion (Cont.)

- **Simultaneous restraint and seclusion:** Patients who are simultaneously restrained and secluded shall by continuously monitored through either face-to-face observation by staff members or remote observation by members located near the patient who are viewing a simultaneous video image and audio signal of the patient.

- **Restraint or seclusion alone:** Patients shall be monitored on an ongoing basis by staff members who are stationed near the patient. The observations made and data collected during such monitoring shall be documented at least every 15 minutes.

- **Assessment:** Assessments by a registered nurse or physician assistant or evaluations by a responsible LIP shall occur as often as indicated by the plan of care based on the patient's condition, behavior, and environmental considerations, but at least once every 60 minutes.

Restraint not used for the management of violent or self-destructive behavior shall be subject to ongoing monitoring and assessment as specified in the patient's plan of care. Monitoring and assessments shall occur at least every two hours.

Discontinuation: Restraint or seclusion shall be discontinued by the registered nurse once the behaviors or situation that served as the basis for the restraint is no longer present and the safety of the patient, staff members, or others may be assured through less restrictive means.

Care plan: The restrained or secluded patient's written plan of care shall be modified to address appropriate interventions implemented to ensure the patient's safety and encourage the prompt discontinuation of restraint.

Reporting restraint-related deaths: Hospital personnel shall promptly contact hospital administration whenever one of the following occurs:

- A patient dies while restrained or within 24 hours after being released from restraint
- A patient dies as the result of a restraint-related condition within seven days after restraint removal
- Hospital administration shall notify CMS of such deaths within one business day of its discovery

Model Policy: Restraint and Seclusion (Cont.)

Training

Hospital and medical staff members shall receive training in the following subjects as appropriate to assigned duties performed under this policy. Such training shall take place before the new staff member is asked to implement the provisions of this policy and shall be repeated periodically as indicated in the hospital's training plan, which shall be based on the results of quality monitoring activities.

Physicians who order restraint or seclusion shall be trained in the requirements of this policy.

Hospital staff members who assess patients for restraint or who apply restraint shall receive training in the following topics as appropriate to the patient population served:

- Techniques to identify staff member and patient behaviors, events, and environmental factors that may trigger circumstances that require the use of a restraint or seclusion

- The use of nonphysical intervention skills

- Choosing the least restrictive intervention based on an individualized assessment of the patient's medical or behavioral status or condition

- The safe application and use of all types of restraint or seclusion by the staff member, including training in how to recognize and respond to signs of physical and psychological distress (e.g., positional asphyxia)

- Clinical identification of specific behavioral changes that indicate that restraint or seclusion is no longer necessary

- Monitoring the physical and psychological well-being of the patient who is restrained or secluded, including but not limited to respiratory and circulatory status, skin integrity, vital signs, and any special requirements specified by hospital policy associated with the one-hour face-to-face evaluation of patients restrained or secluded for the management of violent or self-destructive behavior

- The use of first-aid techniques and certification in the use of cardiopulmonary resuscitation, including required periodic recertification

Hospital staff members who monitor restrained patients shall be trained in the recognition of signs of physical and psychological distress, including the signs of asphyxia.

Standard and Element of Performance	Intent
PC.03.05.03 EP 2	When restraints are initiated, update the patient's care plan.

Even though restraints should have been added to a patient's care plan, the requirement to do so was not specifically stated, as it is now. There are no magic solutions to resolving the struggle we continue to have regarding care planning and updating as changes occur.

Standard and Element of Performance	Intent
PC.03.05.05 EP 3	If an order for restraint or seclusion is obtained from a physician caring for the patient other than the attending physician, the attending physician is to be notified as soon as possible.

To avoid this extra step, it would be best to seek the attending physician for the order, if possible. The EP does not define "as soon as possible." See the definition in the sample policy provided earlier. Defining this with a rigid time frame could set you up for a finding of not following your own policy. It should go without saying that physician notification is to be documented in the medical record.

Standard and Element of Performance	Intent
PC.03.05.05 EP 6	Hospital policy defines the order renewal process for patients restrained for nonviolent or non-self-destructive purposes.

This constitutes a major change, but think this through very carefully as you do not want to revert to bad habits of restraining patients and not carefully considering whether they meet criteria to warrant continuing the restraint. The suggested wording in the sample policy allows the use of a criteria-driven protocol or a time-limited order.

Standard and Element of Performance	Intent
PC.03.05.09 EP 1	Hospital policy is to include the time frames for assessing and monitoring patients in restraint or seclusion.

Because of the risks involved in restraint usage, the sample policy continues to include reasonable time frames for patient monitoring. Compare these to your current policy. Hospitals have often set such rigid monitoring requirements that the patient is not benefiting from the frequency, and the documentation is a page full of hash marks, which is a waste of valuable patient care time.

Standard and Element of Performance	Intent
PC.03.05.09 EP 2	LIPs who are authorized to order restraints are to have a working knowledge of the hospital's policy.

Before you agonize over how to accomplish this task, step back a moment and think about what "working knowledge" really means. It would be nearly impossible for a physician practicing in a hospital not to be able to articulate the basic components of restraint usage. The EP does not require a formalized educational process, so do not go down that road as it will be ineffective. Instead, consider the following "cheat sheet" of general information.

Elsewhere Medical Center

PHYSICIAN INFORMATION

Restraint and Seclusion

Physicians and other licensed independent practitioners (LIP) are required to have a "working knowledge" of <<name of hospital>> policy on restraint and seclusion. Here are the salient points from the restraint and seclusion policy:

Definitions

Restraint is any manual method, physical or mechanical device, material, or equipment that immobilizes or reduces the ability of a patient to move his or her arms, legs, body, or head freely.

Seclusion is the involuntary confinement of a patient alone in a room or an area from which he or she is physically prevented from leaving.

Chemical restraint is the use of a medication to restrict a patient's freedom of movement that is not a standard treatment for the patient's new or continuing medical or behavioral condition. It is this hospital's policy to only use medications that are a standard treatment for the patient's ongoing or newly emerging condition. Therefore, chemical restraint is not used in this institution.

Elsewhere Medical Center (Cont.)

Restraint or seclusion is assessment-driven and is implemented only when it is deemed necessary to protect the physical safety of patients, staff members, or others *and* less restrictive measures have been considered and/or attempted and have been found to be ineffective. Seclusion may be used for management of violent or self-destructive behavior that jeopardizes the immediate safety of the patient, a staff member, or others.

Ordering

Restraint to protect the patient from self-injury and to promote healing (prevention of dislodging of ET tube, lines, etc.) must be ordered by an LIP with a RENEWAL order every calendar day based on the LIP's evaluation of the patient. *If a protocol is used, the restraint order remains in effect until the patient no longer exhibits the behaviors that justified restraint for self-protection.

A registered nurse may initiate restraints and obtain an order from an LIP who is responsible for the patient as soon as possible after restraint is initiated.

The attending physician must be notified as soon as possible (this can be done through review of the restraint order), but no later than the end of the calendar day following initiation of the restraint order, if he or she was not the LIP initiating the restraint.

Restraint or seclusion orders for violent and/or self-destructive behavior that jeopardizes the immediate safety of a patient, a staff member, or others shall remain in effect until the patient's behavior or situation no longer requires the use of restraint or seclusion, but no longer than:

- Four hours for adults 18 years of age or older
- Two hours for children and adolescents 9–17 years of age
- One hour for children 8 years of age or younger

Renewal orders may be given for the preceding durations if the indications for restraint or seclusion persist. However, continuation of restraint or seclusion for longer than 24 hours shall be based on an in-person evaluation by a responsible LIP.

One-hour face-to-face assessment: A responsible LIP, a registered nurse, or a physician assistant shall perform a face-to-face assessment of the patient's physical and psychological status within one hour of the initiation of restraint or seclusion.

> **Elsewhere Medical Center (Cont.)**
>
> **PRN orders:**
> PRN orders for restraint or seclusion are *not* to be used.
>
> Exceptions: A standing or PRN order may be used for the following interventions:
>
> - The patient requires the use of a Geri chair with the tray locked to be safety out of bed
> - Bed side rails are used as a restraint (refer to Attachment A)
> - Interventions are used to protect the patient from repetitive self-mutilating behavior
>
> If any LIP has any questions regarding <<name of hospital>> policy on restraint or seclusion, please contact <<name of quality/risk manager or medical staff coordinator or other contact person>> at hospital extension xxxx.

Standard and Element of Performance	Intent
PC.03.05.13 EP 1	Continuous monitoring either in person by a trained staff member or with the use of both audio and video equipment is to occur when a patient is simultaneously restrained and secluded.

There are no shortcuts to this very important patient safety activity. Staff members assigned to monitor the patient must be thoroughly trained and capable of intervening, should the need arise.

Standard and Element of Performance	Intent
PC.04.01.01 EP 23, EP 24, and EP 25	When discharge plans include home healthcare or post-hospital extended care, the list of available agencies is documented in the plan. Documentation includes the provision of the listing to the patient and the disclosure of financial interests between the hospital and the agency.

Often, discharge planners use the listing of possible agencies and facilities as a worksheet and do not include it as a permanent part of the patient's record. Because the EPs were drafted from *CoPs*, they are applicable to Medicare providers. Hospital discharge planners have verbalized their intent to apply the requirements to all patients, regardless of their payer source.

Standard and Element of Performance	Intent
RC.02.01.01 EP 2	All orders are included in the revised listing of elements to be contained within the patient's medical record.

When care is provided in accordance with a protocol, a copy of the protocol should be entered into the patient's medical record. This can also occur with electronic records via document scanning. The record is supposed to tell the "story of care." Should a record be pulled for retrospective review, missing protocols, and therefore orders, increases the hospital's liability for safe care.

Standard and Element of Performance	Intent
RC.02.01.03 EP 15	A complete and up-to-date surgical log is to be maintained.

Ten elements are to be included in the log: patient's name, patient's age, patient's hospital identification number, surgery date, procedure performed, total surgical time, names of surgeon and assistants, names of nursing personnel, type of anesthesia and provider's name, and pre- and postoperative diagnoses. Hospitals with manual operating room records may have continued the laborious task of recording these elements into a daily log book. If at all possible, work with your health information departments to abstract and generate electronic reports. Test the reports to validate that all elements are present. You must present this log during a CMS survey, so it is reasonable to expect that The Joint Commission may also begin requesting it.

Noncompliance at a CMS Condition Level

With the cross-referencing and alignment of the Joint Commission standards to the CMS *CoPs*, there is also an increased expectation that surveyors will identify when there is noncompliance at the CMS condition level. Often, this is referred to as a "condition out." This represents a significant change in The Joint Commission's survey process. At a recent session of Executive Briefings, *CoP* condition out was a topic of discussion. Here are excerpts from the presentation:

There has always been an obligation for The Joint Commission to notify CMS when a condition out was identified and to perform a follow-up survey after the condition was corrected. However, it was stated that most surveyors were not fully cognizant of this issue. Rarely was

Addressing the Changes in Standards for 2009

this a problem for healthcare organizations (except for home care, where this happened more frequently). With the recent alignment of standards with CMS CoPs, if a surveyor identifies a "condition-level finding" there will be a resurvey by The Joint Commission of that condition within 90 days following the 10-day clarification period. When there is a condition out, the surveyor's report will go to the Central Office for review and scoring.

- *A condition out does not always equal conditional accreditation, unless the hospital was also found to be in conditional accreditation pursuant to the Joint Commission standards during the survey*
- *Only The Joint Commission returns for the follow-up visit; not the CMS delegated Department of Health*
- *Extensive surveyor training regarding the CMS CoPs has occurred*
- *Organizations will be charged for the follow-up visit*

To solidify that changes are forthcoming regarding CMS, the October 2009 issue of *Perspectives* included a sample of a "Summary of CMS Findings." A new document that will be incorporated into The Joint Commission's survey report, this summary provides a helpful crosswalk to the corresponding CMS regulations and assists the reader by indicating whether the finding is at the CMS standards or condition level. For accreditation specialists who are still on a learning curve for digesting the *CoPs*, this will be most helpful.

The following standards changes were also published in the October 2009 issue of *Perspectives*:

Standard and Element of Performance	Intent
LD.04.03.09 EP 9 MS.13.01.01 EP 1	For hospitals utilizing the Joint Commission accreditation for deemed status purposes, all physicians are to be credentialed and privileged at the originating site, which is the site where the patient is located.

Hospitals that utilize telemedicine for interpretation of radiology exams, fetal monitoring, and other externally provided medical services previously had the option of accepting the credentialing of the telemedicine practitioners from a Joint Commission–accredited entity.

This was an advantage to the hospital where the patient was located because of the large volume of physicians who might rotate call and provide interpretive services that vary from day to day; the medical staff office could exempt them from their labor-intensive internal credentialing and privileging process as a component of a contracted service. Effective July 15, 2010, all practitioners providing care, services, and treatment must be credentialed and privileged by the hospital.

The Joint Commission must survey to the CMS requirements, but it continues to pursue discussions with CMS and members of Congress to promote the use of credentialing and privileging by proxy. If ever there was a time for your hospital and medical staff leaders to get involved, this is it. If we place this undue burden onto hospitals, particularly smaller rural hospitals that greatly benefit from telemedicine, patients will ultimately suffer as the services will be too costly to support. Encourage your leaders to speak with hospital associations and medical societies about this issue.

Standard and Element of Performance	Intent
LD.04.04.05 EP 13 PI.01.01.01 EP 2	EP 13: Annually, the governing body is to be informed of a specific number of patient safety improvement projects to be conducted. EP 2: The frequency and detail of data collection are specified by the governing body.

You can meet these requirements by integrating them into the prioritization process that is already required in LD.04.04.01. Keep it simple by listing the projects in an annual work plan that is presented to the governing body for approval as part of the performance improvement plan evaluation. A simple tool such as the one displayed in Figure 2.1 will assist you in meeting these two new requirements.

Standard and Element of Performance	Intent
RI.01.07.01 EP 18	The written notice provided to the individual who lodged the complaint is to include the following information: name of the hospital contact person, what investigative steps were taken, results, and when the complaint process was completed.

A thorough complaint and grievance process has always been a priority with CMS, and so now it may also be in the spotlight during the Joint Commission surveys. If you have utilized CMS requirements in formulating your current process, you may have already included these items. Figure 2.2 provides a sample letter for you to use as reference.

Figure 2.1 — Hospitalwide Performance Improvement Annual Workplan

Activity	Indicator(s)	Goal	Data Summary	Responsible Person(s)
Critical Results –Physician Notification	% of critical results called to the physician within one hour of identifying the critical result	100%	Monthly	Directors from Radiology, Lab, and Cardiology Report Quarterly to the Patient Safety Committee
		Sample		

Figure 2.2 ■ Letter for Completion of Grievance Investigation

Dear [*Grievant Name*]:

Subject: Grievance Number NNNN

[*General nature of complaint (e.g. nursing care, food, discharge concerns)*]

We finished our investigation of your concern on [*Date*].

Here is a brief description of what we did to look into the matter:

[*Brief explanation of how you investigated the matter*]

We have taken the following steps aimed at resolving the situation.

[*Brief explanation of what you intend to do to address the issue*]

We feel that this resolution is appropriate and reasonable. However, if you disagree or if there are further things you would like to discuss, please contact our Patient Advocate, <<NAME>>, at <<NUMBER>>. We have attached a copy of our admission packet that includes other information about the complaint and grievance process.

Very truly yours,

[*Name*]

Attachment:

Excerpt from patient admission packet addressing the Patient Complaint and Grievance process.

TEST YOUR KNOWLEDGE

1. True or false: Organizations with off-site patient care services are required to provide each location with a crash cart with appropriate emergency supplies.

Answer: False. Medical staff policies and procedures are required to define the initial treatment and referral of patient emergencies. Interventions should be determined appropriate to the provided care. A crash cart is one option, but so are CPR and 911.

2. Which of the following is correct regarding the requirements for a post-anesthesia evaluation?
- A. An anesthesia provider may delegate the evaluation to a trained PACU nurse
- B. Evaluations are to be performed immediately after surgery or a procedure requiring anesthesia/moderate sedation
- C. The medical staff is to approve the post-anesthesia evaluation policy and procedure
- D. An evaluation performed in the PACU for a patient who received spinal anesthesia is acceptable

Answer: C. An individual who is qualified to administer anesthesia is to perform the anesthesia. The remaining answers are incorrect because delegation to a nurse is unacceptable; an evaluation is not required after the administration of moderate sedation, and instead is to occur within 48 hours to assess recovery from anesthesia; and a patient who received spinal anesthesia would not have fully recovered while in the PACU.

3. Multiple standard changes regarding the use of restraints and seclusion were issued March 26, 2009. Regarding those changes, all of the following statements are true except for one. Can you identify the false statement?
- A. Restraints may be ordered by a physician or other authorized licensed independent practitioner
- B. Violent or self-destructive behavioral restraints are synonymous with the previous terminology of protective restraints
- C. Orders are renewed for nonviolent or non-self-destructive patients as defined in the hospital's policy
- D. Physicians and other licensed independent practitioners are to have a working knowledge of the hospital's restraint policy

Answer: B. Prior to the release of the March 26, 2009, revised standards, the Joint Commission terminology was "restraints for behavioral health purposes." The new term is now the same for both CMS and The Joint Commission.

CHAPTER 3

Frequently Cited Standards and How to Avoid Them

Through my work with hospitals across the country, I hear certain standards that continue to be cited over and over again. In many cases, the hospital has established a policy or procedure that exceeds the intent of the elements of performance (EP). When staff performance does not comply with the organization's requirements, the surveyor finds the EP noncompliant, which subsequently yields the standard noncompliant. In the surveyor's written report, these types of findings are typically explained as follows:

> *Identified during tracer activity in the medical unit, the hospital's policy regarding ... was not followed.*

In this chapter, we will explore various topics that have been overinterpreted and whose bar of expectations has been raised too high. I will also provide simplified policies and documents when applicable.

Issue 1: Failure to Check Crash Carts at the Frequency Required by the Organization's Policy

Interestingly, no standard or EP requires an organization to even check a crash cart. Let's look at the EPs that are commonly cited when this procedural deviation is identified:

- **MM.03.01.03 EP 2:** In patient care areas, emergency medications and associated supplies are readily available.

- **PC.02.01.11 EP 2:** Based on the patient population, resuscitation equipment is available for use.

Chapter 3

- **EC.02.04.01 EP 3 and EP 4:** An inventory of medical equipment, including all life support equipment, is maintained. Inspection and testing for equipment in the inventory are identified in writing.

- **LD.04.01.07 EP 2:** Policies and procedures are implemented.

Missing from this list is any requirement for a crash cart check or a documentation log. It seems that for years, hospitals have performed crash cart checks from frequencies of daily to once per shift. Probably somewhere in the nation, a defibrillator was needed and it malfunctioned. In response, hospitals implemented an over-reactive process to double-check the checker. Repetitive processes without findings tend to generate complacency and shortcuts.

Some hospitals have even established a policy that once per month the cart will be opened and a complete inventory will be performed to ensure that the cart is intact even though the breakaway lock is intact and the number on the breakaway lock has remained the same the entire month. Within the same facilities, I have observed variations in practice between patient care areas. And what happens when the unit is closed for weekends or low census? The log for documenting the cart checks is blank for the closed dates, making it look like those dates were missed.

If any of this sounds familiar, read on and consider reevaluating your organization's process.

Key Concept

The intent is to have emergency medications and supplies readily available. This begins with stocking the cart at setup and after each use. Rethink what actions are required to ensure that the cart is maintained.

When the breakaway lock number does not change, the contents of the cart are intact. Affix to the cart the date of the next expiring medication and supply. If the dates are not yet met, then items are current. Ask your biomedical department to supply the manufacturer's recommendations for testing the function of the defibrillator or AED used in specified units. Some models self-check and others display a light when the battery is fully charged, and they may not need some of the current checks as long as the battery is fresh. Assign the responsibilities for ensuring that these steps are being followed to a person such as the charge nurse or lead technician in ancillary departments.

This process is similar to ensuring that adequate staffing or necessary equipment is available, so why do we require documentation? We don't document that we have locked the narcotics cabinet; we just do it.

If you still choose to use a documentation log, ensure that closed days are documented. Also, keep the current log available only for recording, and file any past logs. There is no need to allow retrospective review if there was a slip in documentation.

Success Story

A hospital that chose to continue documenting the readiness of its crash cart established a policy that the cart would be checked daily on the days that the patient care unit was operational. The hospital's procedure was to check the cart each 12-hour shift. That way, if staff members missed a shift check, they would still be in compliance with their policy of daily checking.

Issue 2: Pain Reassessments Not Performed in Accordance with Hospital Policy

With the advent of pain management and the emphasis on a patient's right to have his or her pain controlled, hospitals reacted by drafting extensive policies that referenced definitions of pain, types of pain, research results on the horrors of not controlling pain, recommendations for analgesics, and so on. And when patient care staff members were interviewed, they were oblivious to the content of this extremely large document.

Here are the four components of standard PC.01.02.07, which deals with pain management:

- **EP 1:** A pain assessment is to be performed in settings where it benefits the patient
- **EP 2:** The assessment tool utilized should take into consideration the patient's age, ability to understand, and condition
- **EP 3:** Based on criteria, there is a response to the patient experiencing pain and a reassessment
- **EP 4:** Pain is treated or a referral is generated

"All" patients need not be assessed for pain. It is not required. It may be prudent to include an initial pain assessment as a component to nursing assessments for emergency department entries or inpatient admissions, but why would a pain assessment be required for patients undergoing routine testing or noninvasive evaluations? Is that not why we employ professionals who are skilled in recognizing the signs and signals of probable pain and then initiate a pain assessment as appropriate to the patient's chief complaint or disease process? Nothing is required regarding establishing a patient-specific pain goal.

This has been driven by hospital policies and is not included in the standards.

Reassessment criteria are to be developed by the hospital and do not require any preassigned frequencies, such as 10 minutes for IV medications, 30 minutes for IM, and one hour for oral medications. These are some of the extremes that can set up a hospital for failure. Sadly, a rigid requirement such as a pain assessment every four hours, whether it is needed or not, is no longer an enhancement to patient care, but is now a burden that robs valuable time from the caregiver. Ask whether your pain assessment practices are geared toward times and frequencies or toward the patient's needs and disease processes.

Do not assume that all patient care providers are familiar with pain assessment tools. Some facilities still use the Wong-Baker FACES Pain Rating Scale to determine a patient's pain level. Unfortunately, such use will result in an inaccurate pain determination. This tool was developed for children who are cognitively developed to a level where they can grasp the concept that they are to point to the face that best represents how they are feeling.

Formulate your policy in a way that allows the caregiver some leeway in determining when a pain assessment should be included in the collection of patient-specific information. Ensure that a pain tool as been selected for assessing pain in patients of all ages, beginning with newborns. Do not forget that an assessment tool is needed for cognitively impaired adults who may be under the influence of sedatives or those who are developmentally impaired.

Should you need some assistance with pain assessment, here is a sample policy and a poster-style listing of pain assessment tools. Additionally, an Internet search of *pain assessment* will yield a large number of tools and sample documents.

Policy Title: Pain Assessment, Reassessment, and Treatment

Department(s): Hospitalwide

Effective Date:

Review Dates:

Scope and Intent

This policy addresses the assessment and reassessment of pain in all settings throughout the organization. When pain is identified, the patient shall be treated or referred for treatment as clinically pertinent.

Policy:

1. Patients admitted as inpatients and presenting to the emergency department shall be questioned as to whether they are experiencing pain. Other ambulatory patients need not be assessed for the presence of pain unless a) pain is commonly associated with the condition for which they are seeking care or b) pain may be induced by subsequent treatments or interactions (e.g., patients undergoing an outpatient invasive procedure or potentially painful therapy).

2. An age- and ability-appropriate comprehensive initial pain assessment shall be conducted for any patient reporting or suspected of having moderate or severe pain. The comprehensive assessment shall include, to the extent relevant, intensity (using an age-appropriate pain scale when practical and available), site(s), quality (e.g., dull, sharp, throbbing, stabbing), radiation, and onset (e.g., the start of the pain and whether it is increasing or decreasing). The details of the initial pain assessment may vary depending on the clinical presentation and the nature of the interaction. For example, a physician's note addressing the patient's pain as part of medical screening or a physical examination is considered a comprehensive pain assessment.

3. A reassessment for the presence and intensity of pain shall be performed as a component of the shift assessment for inpatients and following any intervention intended to lessen the patient's pain (e.g., administration of pain medications, application of cold packs, repositioning).
    a. Such reassessment shall take place within a clinically appropriate time frame, depending on the type of intervention and the route of medication administration.
    b. The caregiver may document the reassessment of a pain intervention at the end of the shift.

4. Patients and, when appropriate, family members, shall be educated in their role(s) in managing pain and the potential limitation and side effect of pain treatments.

Figure 3.1 ■ Pain Assessment Tools

Scale A₁ English

Please point to the number that best describes your pain.

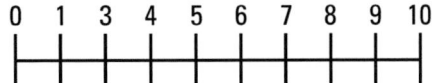

Scale A₁ Spanish

Por favor senale al numero que mejor describe su dolor (Mas grande el numero mayor su dolor).

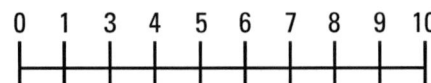

Scale B (PAINAD)

Breathing	Negative Vocalization	Facial Expression	Body Language	Consolability
Normal (0)	None (0)	Smiling/inexpressive (0)	Relaxed (0)	No need to console (0)
Labored (1)	Occasional moans or muttering (1)	Sad/frown (1)	Tense/pacing (1)	Distracted/reassurable (1)
Noisy/extended Cheyne-Stokes respirations (2)	Repeated troubled calling out or loud moaning or crying (2)	Facial grimacing (3)	Rigid with fists clenched/striking out (2)	Unable to distract or reassure (2)

Total _____ = 0–10 pain scale

Scale C Wong-Baker

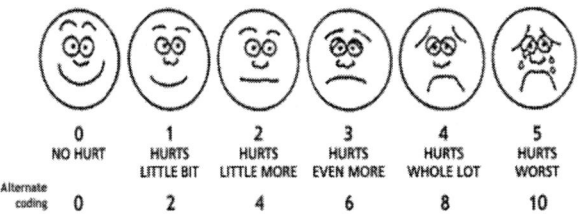

Scale D (<3 years)

Face	0 – No particular expression or smile 1 – Occasional grimace or frown, withdrawn, disinterested 2 – Frequent to constant frown, clenched jaw, quivering chin
Legs	0 – Normal position or relaxed 1 – Uneasy, restless, tense 2 – Kicking, or legs drawn up
Activity	0 – Lying quietly, normal position, moves easily 1 – Squirming, shifting back and forth, tense 2 – Arched, rigid, or jerking
Cry	0 – No cry (awake or sleep) 1 – Moans or whimpers, occasional complaint 2 – Crying steadily, screams or sobs, frequent complaints
Consolibility	0 – Content, relaxed 1 – Reassured by occasional touching, hugging, or "talking to," distractible 2 – Difficult to console or comfort

Figure 3.1 ■ Pain Assessment Tools (Cont.)

Neonatal/Infant Pain Scale (NIPS)

(Recommended for children less than 1 year old.) A score greater than 3 indicates pain.

Facial Expression	
0 – Relaxed muscles	Restful face, neutral expression
1 – Grimace	Tight facial muscles; furrowed brow, chin, jaw, (negative facial expression—nose, mouth, and brow)
Cry	
0 – No Cry	Quiet, not crying
1 – Whimper	Mild moaning, intermittent
2 – Vigorous Cry	Loud scream; rising, shrill, continuous (**Note:** Silent cry may be scored if baby is intubated as evidenced by obvious mouth and facial movement.
Breathing Patterns	
0 – Relaxed	Usual pattern for this infant
1 – Change in Breathing	Indrawing, irregular, faster than usual; gagging; breath holding
Arms	
0 – Relaxed/Restrained	No muscular rigidity; occasional random movements of arms
1 – Flexed/Extended	Tense, straight legs; rigid and/or rapid extension, flexion
Legs	
0 – Relaxed/Restrained	No muscular rigidity; occasional random leg movement
1 – Flexed/Extended	Tense, straight legs; rigid and/or rapid extension, flexion
State of Arousal	
0 – Sleeping/Awake	Quiet, peaceful sleeping or alert random leg movement
1 – Fussy	Alert, restless, and thrashing

Issue 3: Updated History and Physical on the Day of Surgery

The starting point for when a history and physical (H&P) is required is outlined in PC.01.02.03 EP 4 and EP 5. Most medical professionals have grasped the concept that within 24 hours of admission, an H&P must be in the record. Medical professionals also tend to know that an H&P that was performed within the preceding 30 days can be utilized. But where people get confused is the update to the standards that concerns when the H&P was performed within the preceding 30 days but *not* on the day of admission or *not* on the day of same-day/outpatient surgery.

> **Key Concept**
>
>
>
> Update records if there were any changes in the patient's condition since the H&P was performed. The H&P could have been done 30, 15, seven, or one day prior to the day of the surgery, but if it was not done on the same day as the procedure, an update is required. Remember: The H&P must be in the patient's record within 24 hours of admission, not within 24 hours of the surgery. Here is an excerpt from the applicable EP to support the requirement:
>
> - PC.01.02.03 EP 5: An H&P exam must be completed within 30 days prior to inpatient admission or registration, and an update must be completed within 24 hours after an inpatient admission or registration, but prior to surgery or a procedure requiring anesthesia, whichever comes first.

We believe The Joint Commission included the word *registration* in the March 26, 2009, version of the standards because folks were still hung up on the "prior to surgery" requirement.

Even if a physician saw the patient less than 24 hours before he or she was admitted, the physician must update the patient's H&P. For example, what if the patient was diabetic, had heart disease, and was scheduled for an exploratory laparotomy? A physician should want to know whether the patient was in the emergency room the preceding night for an episode of low blood sugar, as that may have an impact on whether the patient is still a candidate for the surgical procedure. And that is the key reason for an update: to state prior to surgery that nothing has changed since the patient was last seen by the physician, and that it is appropriate to proceed with the procedure.

> **Success Stories**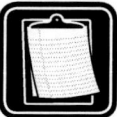
>
> "Stop! H&P Update." As physicians came to the holding area to see the patient, they would see the sign and ask the patient, "Has anything changed since I last saw you?" If nothing had changed, the physicians would write "No changes" and would sign the chart, as well as note the date and time they met with the patient.
>
> At another facility, the medical staff included in their rules and regulations that the preanesthesia evaluation performed on the day of surgery would serve as the update to the surgeon's H&P. This is a perfectly acceptable solution.

Issue 4: Requiring an H&P Prior to Moderate Sedation

First, it is important to state that no standard/EP requires an H&P prior to moderate sedation. The Centers for Medicare & Medicaid Services (CMS) also does not require it because it addresses issues that occur prior to anesthesia, and moderate sedation is not anesthesia.

Second, other than the requirements discussed in the preceding section, MS.03.01.01 EP 6 clearly gives the power to the medical staff to specify the minimal content of an H&P and to state when an H&P is required based on the level of patient care and the setting.

Offer the medical staff a sample of a focused H&P to be used prior to invasive procedures that are of moderate risk to the patient and whose content considers the functions of the heart and lung and whatever else the proceduralist believes is pertinent to the safe care of that particular patient. Also, remember that nothing prevents a nurse and physician from working as a team, with the nurse completing the history and the physician completing the physical.

> **Key Concept**
>
> Prepare a list of procedures performed outside the operating room that tend to produce questions regarding whether an H&P is required. Involve several physicians from, perhaps, interventional radiology and a specialty that performs a large portion of their procedures as outpatients, such as an otolaryngologist. Have this list approved by the medical staff leaders, typically the medical executive committee. Keep the approved list handy and follow what was recommended. A physician or nurse can always collect additional information if the situation warrants it, but a shortcut is a surefire invitation for a patient safety occurrence or a citation of noncompliance.

Located in Appendix A.6 of this book is an example of a table created with a client to serve as a ready reference for physicians and staff members performing procedures outside the operating room. It contains additional information such as what component of the Universal Protocol™ is required, whether a formal post-procedure note is required versus a progress note entry, and other items beyond the H&P requirements. With the changes in the Universal Protocol, the document may need updating, so consider the concept of the tool and not the contents.

Issue 5: Untimely Primary Source Verification of Practitioner and Staff Licenses

Medical staff offices have been required to do this for years, but only in the past several years has this been pulled over to the Human Resources chapter, and the transition has not been smooth in all facilities. The standard that drives primary source verification for employees is HR.01.02.05. EP 1 states that when laws or regulations require the patient care provider to be licensed, certified, or registered to practice, the hospital must verify that there is a current license, certification, or registration from the entity that issues such credentials (primary source verification), and must document that the verification has occurred. (Within this section, I will use the term *license*, but you should consider it to also include registration and certification.)

Primary source verification has to occur at the time of hire and as the credential is renewed. And here is the rub: The verification must occur before the individual practices in your facility and again before his or her credential expires at midnight on the expiration date. In other words, if you are using the

Internet to verify a credential, the date on the bottom of the print version must be before the credential expires.

And let's not forget that The Joint Commission may go back to any activities that have occurred subsequent to its last on-site survey. Therefore, do *not* destroy the evidence that primary source verification has occurred. The activity must be documented. If this has not occurred, noncompliance will be cited. (See Appendix A.6b on this book' accompanying Web site for a helpful Verbal Verification Form.)

Field Experience

Facilities that have decentralized primary source verification have more issues with this requirement than those that maintain a centralized responsibility with the human resources department. This is a time-sensitive requirement, and therefore it requires a mechanism to alert the individual responsible for primary source verification that it is time to once again verify. In some states, all licenses within a specific profession expire at the same time. In other states, they expire on the individual's expiration date. Regardless, organizations must have some sort of a tickler system to manage primary source verification in a timely manner.

Key Concept

Exchange the time your organization is spending to collect copies of licenses with primary source verification via the Internet or telephone calls to agencies not offering online verification. The EP does *not* require a copy of the credential. Savvy computer whizzes are able to duplicate some credentials and The Joint Commission does not want to see the paper copy. It wants to know that the agency responsible for issuing the license has indeed done so. In addition, when verification is obtained, not only do you receive information that the license is current, but you also receive information regarding any action on the license. If you have employees moonlighting at other facilities and for some reason an action has occurred against their license, you will obtain this information.

Success Story

A hospital struggling to get its arms around this required activity researched the use of a credentials verification organization (CVO) to perform primary source verification for its licensed personnel. Hospital personnel were pleasantly surprised at the inexpensive cost and the fact that once they provided the CVO with the employee's name, the CVO tracked the expiration data and provided the primary source verification to the hospital before expiration. The burden was removed from the human resources department and the managers throughout the organization. Best of all, they were in compliance. In addition, some CVOs will concurrently monitor a state's license action reports and notify you should one of your employees have an action posted against his or her license. This is a service that is well worth looking into.

Key Concept

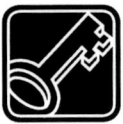

If you choose to obtain primary source verification over the phone, documentation is crucial. Insufficient documentation of telephone verification will result in a finding of noncompliance.

Before we leave this topic, I should note that EP 2 under the same human resources standard requires the hospital to verify, *not* necessarily via primary source verification, a license, registration, or certification that is not required by law and regulation but is required by the hospital. Your method of verification may be a letter or card that displays successful completion of advanced cardiac life support (ACLS) or it could be a letter from a certification board that the applicant is not eligible for board certification if this is a requirement for the position. Examples could be ACLS certification, certification as an infection control practitioner, and so forth. These items are typically listed in job descriptions under the title "Qualifications" and again are required by the hospital. If you require certifications at the time of hire, you must have a method for verifying that certification must occur before the employee begins work. And again, the process must be documented.

Issue 6: Inadequate Monitoring of Contracted Clinical Services

The standard LD.04.03.09 has been around for several years, but it is still not impressing upon administrative leaders the fact that The Joint Commission means business when clinical services are contracted to an external entity. Compliance with this standard really begins at the time of contract. As an accreditation specialist, you may not know that leaders are considering outsourcing a service until staff members appear and announce, "Hi, I am from ABC Dialysis." At this point, EP 2, which describes the scope of services, and EP 4, which establishes expectations for performance of the contracted services would be a done deal.

Field Experience

One thing that might help you avoid this pitfall is to work with the administrative assistant who is "in the know" regarding contracted services and usually works within the C-suite. Ask that an inventory of contracted clinical services be formulated. This information will likely be asked at the beginning of your on-site survey, so you might as well be tracking it now. Perform a gap analysis of each contracted clinical service to ensure that the EPs within standard LD.04.03.09 have been met; if they haven't, initiate contract addenda to fill in the identified gaps. Most contracted services are involved with multiple hospitals, so this should not be a surprise to them. If you need it at your hospital, chances are good that they have already experienced this requirement at other hospitals.

To assist your organization in evaluating contracted clinical services, the checklist in figure 3.2 could be helpful.

Figure 3.2 ■ Contracted Clinical Services Checklist

Contracted Entity _____ Date Initiated _____

Responsible Individual _____

Method to Evaluate Performance _____
_____
_____

Contract includes: (check off as applicable)

- ❏ Clinical leaders and medical staff had an opportunity to provide advice about the sources of clinical services provided through contract (EP 1)
- ❏ The written contract contains the nature and scope of services provided by the contractor (EP 2)
- ❏ Designated leader(s) approved the contract (EP 3)
- ❏ The contract describes the expectations of performance as a basis to evaluate the services to determine whether they are being provided in accordance with the contract and at a safe/quality level (EP 4 and 5)
- ❏ Evaluation of contractual performance has occurred by the method described above (EP 6)
- ❏ When performance has not met contractual expectations, steps were taken by the responsible party to improve contractual services (EP 7)
- ❏ Contract requires the contractor to utilize qualified staff to provide services; definition of qualified may need to be defined by the vendor in collaboration with the hospital (HR.01.06.01 EP 1)
- ❏ Contract includes language that the contractor will abide by all the Joint Commission standards (Introduction of LD.04.03.09: The same level of care should be delivered …)

Date Contract Evaluated _____

Evaluator _____

Issue 7: Deviation from High-Level Disinfection Procedures

> **Field Experience**
>
>
> Your survey is going along great. The infection control session went without a hitch. Then the surveyors entered the ultrasound suite and saw a container on the counter. They asked the technician, "What is in the container?" and the technician replied, "That is how we clean our vaginal ultrasound probes." And then the questions began: What product is being used? How long is the solution effective? How do you test the efficacy? Can I see the testing log? How do you know when it is time to change the disinfectant? How were you trained to use high-level disinfection techniques? Who else is competent to manage this high-level disinfection process?

To avoid this trap and to ensure that high-level disinfection is accomplishing true disinfection, prepare an inventory of every location where high-level disinfection is occurring. If you cannot compile a thorough list of where the procedure is being performed, you can't correct this potential problem.

Engage your infection control staff to assist with this endeavor. In the October 2009 issue of *Perspectives*, edits to the infection control standard IC.02.02.01 were published. The lead article supports the fact that identified problems with high-level disinfection with endoscopes have led to increased scrutiny of the sterilization and disinfection of medical equipment. The contents of the article are beyond the scope of this book, but it is critical that you read the article in its entirety and follow the recommendations it outlines.

> **Key Concept**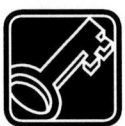
>
> While you're formulating an inventory of locations where high-level disinfection is utilized, visit the department and enlist their assistance in responding to the questions mentioned in the preceding Field Experience sidebar. There is no wiggle room with EP 2. It is a category A EP. Ask which personnel have been trained and how competency was assessed. Determine where such competency is documented. Subsequently, select several staff members and ask that documentation be provided. Consider this a "mock" infection control tracer so that you get the attention of the departments *and* report the findings at the infection control committee meeting. If actions are needed to bring the practice into compliance, formulate an action plan and report progress to the committee until resolution is achieved. Be sure to report any findings of noncompliance to the Joint Commission steering committee so that the item can be entered into the committee's organizationwide compliance monitoring.

Issue 8: Missing or Incomplete Physician Orders

Frequently, our clients ask us where The Joint Commission and CMS stand in terms of standing orders, protocols, preprinted order sets, and orders in general, as well as what individual states, especially licensing boards, expect for physician orders prior to carrying out patient care by licensed caregivers.

Much of the confusion around this topic began after CMS updated its *Conditions of Participation (CoP)* in April 2008 with inclusion of the following statement:

> *482.23(c)(2) With the exception of influenza and pneumococcal polysaccharide vaccines, which may be administered per physician-approved hospital policy after an assessment of contraindications, orders for drugs and biologicals must be documented and signed by a practitioner who is authorized to write orders by hospital policy and in accordance with State law, and who is responsible for the care of the patient as specified under 482.12(c).*

The following note[1] was also included:

> *Note: If a hospital uses other written protocols or standing orders for drugs or biologicals that have been reviewed and approved by the medical staff, initiation of such protocols or standing orders requires an order from a practitioner responsible for the patient's care.*

The Joint Commission entered the discussion because the CMS "note" would preclude the use of protocols for rapid response teams and other emergency care. On October 24, 2008, CMS issued a memo removing the "note" and adding the following information:

> *We concluded that the note may cause confusion about the ability of rapid response teams and other health care professionals in hospitals to initiate effective responses to emergency situations and/or to implement best practices for providing necessary patient care in a timely fashion under the aegis of standing orders.*

> *The use of standing orders must be documented as an order in the patient's medical record and authenticated by the practitioner responsible for the care of the patient as the regulations at 42CFR 482.23.(c)(2) and 482.24(c)(1) require, but the timing of such documentation should not be a barrier to effective emergency response, timely and necessary care or other patient safety advances. We would expect to see that the standing order had been entered into the order entry section of the patient's medical record as soon as possible after implementation of the order (much like verbal orders would be entered), with authentication by the patient's physician.*

The memo goes on to address protocols and preprinted order sets and adds to the confusion such terminology as clinical guidelines and standards of practice, but unfortunately does not provide their definitions. One of the most important statements was the following:

> *While there is significant merit to the use of standing orders, there is also the potential for harm to patients if hospitals use such orders so that nurses or other clinical staff are routinely expected to make clinical decisions outside their scope of practice. This is a complex issue which requires careful consideration by hospitals, physicians, nurses and other licensed health care professions, experts in patient safety and quality improvement and patients.*

---

1. For your reference, the entire CMS memo is included in this book's online appendix.

This statement should be instrumental in telling hospitals to explore their state's licensing regulations for the involved professions, not forgetting the pharmacy regulations for ordering and administering medications, as well as the Department of Health regulations for hospital licensing. If these resources are silent and do not address the use of standing orders or protocols implemented without a physician order, the organization must develop its own approach, keeping in mind the critical component of scope of practice with included competency.

The CMS memo included a comment that within "the next several months" CMS would be formulating specific steps and partnerships necessary to accomplish the goals of understanding best practices and the use of various order types. Additional information was not available at the time of this writing.

The following is a recap of the Joint Commission standards/EPs that hinge on the issue of order types (the following recap is paraphrased; see your standards manual for the complete EPs):

- **MM.05.01.07 EP 5:** In accordance with law and regulation, medications are prepared and administered in accordance with the orders of a licensed independent practitioner (LIP); this was added in March 2009 to comply with the same standard from CMS 482.23(c).

- **PC.02.01.03 EP 1, EP 2, and EP 3:** The hospital obtains or renews orders from an LIP prior to providing care, treatment, or services (EP 1). The most recent patient order is used (EP 2). The orders of a doctor are required for providing respiratory services and the services are provided in accordance to the order (EP 3).

- **PC.01.02.15 EP 1:** As ordered, diagnostic tests and procedures are performed.

- **RC.02.01.01 EP 2 (thirteenth bullet point):** All orders are contained in the medical record.

So where do you begin?

1. Research your state's licensing board requirements, practice acts, Department of Health's licensing requirements, and so forth. If your research yields limited results, go to step 2 and consider enlisting the assistance of your legal advisor.

2. Create organizational definitions of order types.

    Through the ages, people pick up on terms and do not change their interpretations of these terms even when the terms' meanings change. Ensure that staff members who state that they utilize "standing orders" are not actually referencing preprinted orders. At a minimum, include the most commonly encountered terms of:

   a. Standing orders

   b. Protocols

   c. Preprinted order sets

3. Provide examples of each order type so that staff members can begin to understand the differences between the order types.

   Use current orders they can relate to, and pull from multiple settings such as the emergency department, intensive care unit, and OPS; don't restrict your work to only nursing. This is an issue for radiology technicians, respiratory therapists, and other patient care staff members as well.

4. Begin the approval process by attaining medical staff input.

   Involving physicians too early in the development process could result in many potentially heated discussions and very few results. Physicians tend to respond more positively when they have a sample document with organizational examples to review.

5. Follow your organization's path to approval, which may include legal review and implementation.

6. Be sure to include education in multiple formats as this could be a major change for some long-term employees.

Field Experience

Because no hard and fast definitions are available for various order types, the following are samples that you might wish to begin with. They have been derived from their use in articles, narrative statements from publications referencing expected practice, and experience from working with multiple hospitals.

Preprinted order sets

A preprinted order set is a menu of listed medications, diagnostic tests, or treatment orders designed around an individual physician's preferences (Dr. Smith's admission orders) or a setting for care (ICU admission orders). Some of the listed orders may require the LIP to adapt dosages or to select the treatments for individual patients depicted by checkboxes and blank fields for data entry.

An order from an LIP must be obtained prior to initiating a preprinted order set. The order may be documented by the LIP with his or her signature, along with the date and time the preprinted order set was obtained, or via a telephone/verbal order documented by the healthcare provider approved to accept telephone/verbal orders.

Preprinted order sets should be reviewed and approved by the medical staff members who will be using the order set. When the order set includes medications, a designated time frame for re-review is to be determined as required in MM.04.01.01 EP 7. It stands to reason that the preprinted order set would become a permanent part of the record.

Protocols

A protocol is a defined, standardized listing of medications, diagnostic tests, or treatments to care for a patient with a specific diagnosis or diagnostic test. A protocol differs from a preprinted order set as a protocol does not include built-in options for selecting patient-specific orders. Variations in weight-based dosing are included in the protocol and the orders are typically derived from evidence-based guidelines.

An order from an LIP is not obtained prior to implementing in emergency situations such as ACLS and hypoglycemia. All other situations require an order. An LIP may provide orders for protocols prior to the occurrence of a symptom so that the nurse is prepared to act should the symptom occur. An example would be an order that reads "Implement chest pain protocol if patient experiences chest pain while in the ICU." Likewise, an order for a pulmonary function test would initiate the protocol to perform the test that may include the administration of a bronchodilator. The same situation could occur for a colonoscopy. A predefined protocol could include the initiation of an IV whenever the LIP gave an order for a colonoscopy.

Protocols are to be approved by the medical staff members who will be using them. A copy of the protocol is to be included in the medical record when it is ordered proactively or when it is implemented in an emergency situation. The implementation of an emergency protocol requires the retrospective signature of an LIP. This ensures that the LIP is aware of the initiation of the protocol and authenticates its use.

Standing orders

A standing order is a prewritten order from an LIP to administer medications, obtain a diagnostic test, or implement a treatment based on a specific symptom. These types of orders differ from preprinted order sets as they are symptom-based with no options to alter the order. They differ from protocols as they are not based on diagnoses and they are implemented in an emergency or routine basis without an LIP order.

Standing orders are approved by the individual practitioner. A copy of the order with the practitioner's signature and approval date is maintained by the patient care department where the order will be utilized.

As the symptom is identified by the caregiver, a copy of the standing order is entered into the order section of the medical record with an entry describing the symptom, the signature of the caregiver initiating the order, and the date and time the order was given.

The signature of an LIP is required to document his or her awareness of the implementation of his or her standing order.

As the reader, you are probably saying, "Wow, we have a lot of work to do." You are not alone in that regard. It seems that hospitals, medical staffs, and patient care providers have allowed practices to develop that may not always be within the scope of their practice and may not always be in the best interests of the patient. This is the hesitation that CMS noted in its memo.

The other problem is the terminology. We need to know what has been approved for use and then call it what it is. I believe that many of the so-called standing orders are actually protocols or preprinted order sets and that the use of standing orders as defined earlier is minimal. With some organizational definitions and productive discussions among the medical staff and patient care providers, this can be turned into a win-win situation for the patient, the LIP, and the caregivers.

CHAPTER 4

Internally Assessing Standards Compliance

Changes are forthcoming regarding the periodic performance review (PPR). The following is a summary of information provided by the speakers at the Joint Commission's Executive Briefings in September 2009:

- A complete revision of the PPR is in process. The torturous process of filling out the PPR will be eliminated as a hospital accreditation requirement; however, the PPR tool will remain on the Joint Commission extranet for organizations that wish to use it for self-assessment purposes.

- There will be a newly defined assessment process that will be mandatory for each organization and will include a feature referenced as "touch points." Touch points were described as time periods (currently proposed at six months and 18 months) in which the organization would have an option of an on-site visit or a telephone call with The Joint Commission. If a telephone call is selected, the organization's account executive and a member of the Standards Interpretation Group (SIG) would represent The Joint Commission. So how would this be structured?

- Six months after the final survey report is posted, The Joint Commission will contact your organization to ensure that the evidence of standards compliance (ESC) and the submitted action plans were implemented and resulted in resolution of noncompliant elements of performance (EP) previously identified during the on-site survey. At that time, The Joint Commission would elicit feedback regarding the survey process, provide an update of the electronic application, and determine the date for the next touch point to occur in 18 months. The option of an on-site visit or telephone call would also be offered for the 18-month touch point.

- During the time between the first touch point and the scheduled second touch point, the organization would be required to complete portions of the PPR that address the structure EPs (primarily the category A EPs), previous problem areas (from previous PPR findings), and organizational risks identified as primary focus areas or data included in the Strategic Surveillance System (S3) score.

- At the 18-month time period, an on-site visit or call with the organization's representative and a member of the SIG would be held where top issues of organizational concern, issues from "like" organizations, top issues from the organization's outcomes data (S3, sentinel events, etc.), implementation ideas, and leading practices that The Joint Commission had gleaned from other organizations would be shared and the electronic application updated, if necessary.

- There would be no charge for the touch point process and it would replace the PPR as it has been known.

- The touch point PPR process would be framed under "shared responsibility for continuously meeting quality standards" and at the time of this writing has not been distributed.

What does this mean to the reader? It means you should change nothing until The Joint Commission prints the official word. If you have specific questions about a PPR that is due fairly soon, contact your account executive and discuss your situation.

Regardless of whether the PPR process changes, the value of performing an internal assessment cannot be underestimated. The concept is not new. While we await the finalization of the PPR requirements, I will reference the PPR as an internal assessment within this chapter.

Whenever procedural changes occur in any industry, the initial step to determining what changes may need to occur is to perform a gap analysis. (Occasionally, I have used that term and people are not familiar with it, so I have provided an official definition in Figure 4.1.)

Internally Assessing Standards Compliance

Figure 4.1 ■ Gap Analysis

Definition:

Technique for determining the steps to be taken in moving from a current state to a desired future state. It begins with (1) listing characteristic factors (such as attributes, competencies, and performance levels) of the present situation ("what is"), (2) cross-listing factors required to achieve the future objectives ("what should be"), and then (3) highlighting the "gaps" that exist and need to be "filled." Also called need-gap analysis, needs analysis, and needs assessment.

You can see that the basics are to determine where you are so that you know where you have to go. Use this approach whenever The Joint Commission publishes a change in requirements.

For managing the paper process and keeping track of the changes as they apply to your organization, as well as for simple changes, print the change and make note of the "gap analysis" on the flip side of the printout.

For more complex changes, use the content of the changes to prepare a table that lists the requirements in one column and your process, document, data collection, and other evidence of compliance in the next column.

In a third column, put a check in the box for compliance versus noncompliance. Figure 4.2 provides a sample gap analysis template. Noncompliant items should then move to the organization's ongoing dynamic action plan for continuous standards compliance, an issue we will discuss in more detail at the end of this chapter and again in Chapter 7.

Key Concept

The following updates are binding in regard to organizations being compliant with standard changes:

- Publishing information in The Joint Commission's *Perspectives*
- Providing memos to the organization on The Joint Commission's Connect extranet
- Posting answers to Frequently Asked Questions on the Joint Commission's Web site

Figure 4.2 ■ Gap Analysis Documentation

Source of new requirements _____

Date received _____ Effective date _____

Gap analysis completed by _____

Date gap analysis completed _____

New Requirement	Evidence of Compliance	Compliance?
		❏ Yes ❏ No
		❏ Yes ❏ No
		❏ Yes ❏ No
		❏ Yes ❏ No
		❏ Yes ❏ No
		❏ Yes ❏ No
		❏ Yes ❏ No
		❏ Yes ❏ No
		❏ Yes ❏ No
		❏ Yes ❏ No
		❏ Yes ❏ No
		❏ Yes ❏ No
		❏ Yes ❏ No
		❏ Yes ❏ No
		❏ Yes ❏ No
		❏ Yes ❏ No

The Joint Commission considers providing these updates to be the equivalent of handing you a newly updated standards manual. At the time this updated information becomes available, assess category A EPs against your defined practice, usually in the form of some type of document, and category C EPs to the implementation of the process. If noncompliance is identified during your gap analysis, immediately add the issues to your continuous compliance action plan and formulate and implement action steps until compliance is achieved.

> **Field Experience**
>
>
>
> Sometimes you may wish to submit an online question to the SIG at The Joint Commission or discuss topics with your account executive. As puzzling as it might seem, these two avenues of assistance are advisory only, and the surveyors are not bound to accept the answers that you receive should they be in conflict with the training the surveyors have had regarding interpretation of standards. It is important to maintain a log of SIG inquiries and your account executive's instructions, as I have found that this type of evidence of trying to do the right thing has been helpful in clarifying Requirements for Improvement (RFI).

Is conducting an internal assessment worth the trouble?

You might already be wondering whether the process is more torturous than it is worth, knowing the time commitments that are required to accomplish the assessment. The No. 1 reason for conducting an internal assessment is to ensure that anytime the organization undergoes an external assessment there will not be any surprises of noncompliance. Leaders should know at all times where the organization is vulnerable to receiving an adverse finding. This process helps to distribute the accountability of standards compliance to others in the organization.

> **Key Concept**
>
>
>
> Leaders and only leaders should make conscious decisions regarding when they are willing to accept noncompliance. If you know there are areas of noncompliance and this is not reported up the chain of command, you are part of the problem and not the solution. This is a tough message, and sometimes it's a tough place to be, but it is a facet of the job of coordinating accreditation readiness. Use the internal assessment process to document noncompliance and disseminate responsibility to others in the organization.

Accreditation specialists should consider the internal assessment to be the first step in achieving continuous survey readiness. Prepare with the end in mind. Consider the documentation that you will need should the EP, and subsequently the standard, be scored as noncompliant in the actual survey. This internal assessment will yield for the organization a wealth of information regarding implementation of required processes, availability of precise policies/procedures that address the key content of EPs, and staff members' understanding of expectations of practice. But before this can happen, leadership must support the assessment process, perhaps exhibited best with their involvement in assessing the leadership chapter and holding line managers accountable to participate in internal assessment efforts.

Most hospitals have either completed an internal self-assessment using their own staff as experts or hired outside consultants to conduct some type of mock survey assessment. Individuals who have been instrumental in facilitating their organization's internal assessment seem to agree that the assessments that dig deep and ask the toughest questions are the most helpful, but are also the most grueling. The comparison of actual practice to written policies, procedures, and guidelines is valuable in determining whether operations are consistent in all care settings and whether patient care delivery can be improved in any way.

> **Field Experience**
>
>
> If a self-assessment is completed around the table based on testimony of attendees or based on memory, you are not digging deep. You must pull the policy or procedure, interview staff members who are doing the work, or observe practices to conduct a valid internal assessment. Based on comments by consultants in the field, there appears to be a correlation between the thoroughness of completing the internal assessment and the results of an organization's triennial survey.

Even the best institutions may identify a significant number of noncompliant EPs, but that is okay. It is the purpose of the exercise. Some of the issues are simple and others will be somewhat complex, but failure to call it what it is, noncompliance, will result in an invalid internal assessment and a waste of time.

Leaders need to support staff members who participate in the internal assessment and let them know that it is okay and expected that issues of noncompliance will "bubble up." Participants need to feel comfortable about being honest and not fear retaliation from management. If managers criticize or indicate displeasure with staff members for exposing deficiencies, the organization's internal assessment will not serve its purpose. This cannot be emphasized enough: If a different outcome is desired (i.e., increased standards compliance), a new way of doing things has to be implemented.

So where do you begin?

Select an Approach to Self-Assessment

If your organization has never conducted a thorough internal assessment as defined by assessing each and every EP and documenting evidence utilized for scoring, you may want to select the chapter approach. If you believe your previous internal assessment met the definition of thorough, your internal assessment may just require a fine-tuning of standards changes and a focus on standards that continue to be problematic in surveys. If so, skip to the focus approach.

Chapter approach

Using the chapters as your guide, persuade an individual to lead the charge for each chapter. Do not get too hung up on the candidates' profession, title, or area of employment because the most important selection criteria are the characteristics of a facilitator, change agent, and attitude regarding accreditation.

Depending on your organizational position and authority, you may be the decision-maker and need not submit a proposed list of chapter leaders to your immediate supervisor. However, if you at least obtain input and share this decision with your organizational leaders, if any grumbling begins within line management, you can draw upon the fact that this process and the chapter leaders were endorsed by hospital leadership. If you choose to skip this step, just be aware that you could end up with the ball in your court and no one to pass to. It takes a team, so build one and use it.

Focused approach

Looking at past survey results, previous internal assessments, and information generated in *Perspectives* regarding the top 10 most problematic standards, select vulnerable processes of care and build your teams around your selection. For example, we know that timely reporting of critical results generated RFIs in 37% of hospitals surveyed in 2008 (as published in the July 2009 issue of *Perspectives*). This may be a vulnerable area for your organization, and a team focused on this topic should be formulated.

Consider all the sites where critical results are defined, generated, and reported: laboratory, radiology, cardiology, respiratory care, emergency department, outpatient clinics, private practitioners, and so forth. Pull a representative from each area to review the reporting of the critical results process—from ordering the test through reporting the critical results to the physician. Don't forget that the process may vary for inpatient versus outpatient procedures/services or patients who were there for testing only. Compare your processes to the required EPs to ensure that the organization is compliant in regard to all sites producing and receiving critical results.

When organizations approach the internal assessment with the use of interdisciplinary focused teams with representatives from all applicable business lines, noncompliance areas are more readily identified and plans of action are implemented to promptly address the issues.

> **Key Concept**
>
>  I cannot emphasize enough the need to assess all patient care areas included in your organization's Joint Commission application. This continues to be an issue with many hospitals that overlook the fact that the off-site wound care center or the recently acquired obstetrics clinic must comply with the hospital standards if they are under the hospital's survey umbrella.

Determine the Scoring Tool to Be Utilized

On the Joint Commission's extranet site, every accredited organization has password-protected access to an electronic PPR tool. There is no charge for this software as it is a component of the accreditation package fees. (Remember, The Joint Commission has reported that this tool will remain available to hospitals even if the requirements of the PPR change.) Enhanced security allows settings to be individualized via the software administrator named at your hospital. All standards and EPs are contained within the software and are specific to your organization's accreditation program(s). The value of using the software is that after scoring each individual EP, the score for the standard is automatically calculated.

Some hospitals have voiced reluctance in using this software because they are concerned about unauthorized access to their data by The Joint Commission or Web site hackers. Entry into the extranet site is password-protected. The facility has control over password assignments and can limit the access rights within various functions to ensure that data are not changed or deleted. Data are not transmitted to The Joint Commission until the Submission key is selected.

In addition to the software storing the EPs and standards scoring, there are free text fields for documenting an action plan, measures of success, and miscellaneous information. A free text area labeled "Miscellaneous Information" is designed for the facility's use only. Data within this area never transmit to The Joint Commission, even when you click the Transmit button.

Field Experience

You could use the miscellaneous field to enter a list of evidence documents used in scoring the EP designated for each standard. The advantage of this is the ability to create references for use during the survey if a surveyor inquires about supporting documents and key persons are not in attendance to answer. These reference materials can be used by anyone who needs to know what was used to score the EPs during the internal assessment. Results of your gap analysis evidence documentation could be added in this software location.

Data entry need not be batched and can occur at the time the EP is being scored. The software contains multiple formatted reports that allow the team to print reports that will identify which standards are noncompliant, which are compliant, which are waiting to be scored, and so forth. The software is a dynamic document and is continuously updated by the internal assessment teams, so at any given time one can view the standards that are scored compliant, are scored noncompliant, and are not scored.

Occasionally, organizations battle with the "owner" of the software, with conflict arising between the hospital software administrator and the internal assessment team leaders who want to be able to manage their team's data entry and reporting. Resolving this conflict just might be the first step toward tearing down those dividing walls that continue to foster silo operations and prevent organizationwide collaboration in working toward standards compliance in *all* departments.

> **Field Experience**
>
>
>
> An internal assessment team leader who can be trusted to lead his or her team through assessment and scoring for such an important job as the Joint Commission accreditation process should be trusted to enter data into a software program. Why hand off a team's scoring to another individual to perform data entry? Isn't it our goal to encourage participation and decentralize the Joint Commission accreditation process? If you answered yes to this question, be instrumental in gaining access to the PPR tool so that team leaders can function efficiently in their roles.

Some organizations have purchased Accreditation Manager Plus software from The Joint Commission. This software functions similarly to the extranet, but the advantage is that it is installed on your organization's shared drive and is managed totally by internal staff members. Should you still need to submit the results of the internal assessment, the data are uploaded to the extranet, so there is no need to perform duplicate data entry.

If your organization works better from hard-copy tools, you can always print the chapters from the extranet. The printed document contains the fields for scoring the individual EPs, and the final standard scoring would occur at the point of data entry. Whatever works best for the style of your organization is acceptable as long as scoring is accurate and thorough.

It Takes a Team: Choose Participants Wisely

Utilize personnel who excelled on teams during previous internal assessments or performance improvement activities. Avoid the naysayers and those who only see problems. During the enhancement to standards compliance, you need creative folks who are eager to see the advantages of trying a process in a different light to achieve compliance.

Keep the team size manageable. A core group of members will be able to score the majority of standards, and it is perfectly acceptable to invite others to participate on an ad hoc basis when setting-specific or topic-specific scoring is needed.

> **Success Story**
>
>
>
> In one hospital, the team leader for medication management was a staff pharmacist. His first task was to utilize the definition of a medication and determine each location in the hospital system where medications were administered. This location list remained visible whenever scoring occurred so that the team would score across the organization and not just think about the most likely department, such as pharmacy or nursing. Because the organization had multiple off-site locations, a member of the core team might be assigned to contact managers off-site to obtain their input prior to finalizing a score. Not only did this improve the team's knowledge of medication management processes in various sites around the organization, but it also improved the validity of scoring organizational compliance.

Provide Education and Training to the Teams

Experiences with the Joint Commission survey process and the nitty-gritty of scoring principles will be varied among team members. And even if they have participated before, the goal is to have accurate scoring that truly represents practices. Therefore, a refresher is warranted.

> **Key Concept**
>
>
>
> Before scoring any EP as not applicable, ensure that inquiries are made to the appropriate organizational staff member. Services change, and the team members may not be aware of all changes. In addition, it is also a good practice to consult with your account executive or possibly submit a question to the SIG if you are unsure whether the EP is applicable. Should the applicability of the EP come up at a later date, this documentation would be available to support your scoring position, even if such documentation is not binding.

One of the most common mistakes individuals make as they begin to self-score is that they do not dissect the entire requirement to understand exactly what is required. As an example, let's use National Patient Safety Goal #15, identifying safety risks inherent in the organization's population. A note attached to the standard states, "This requirement applies only to psychiatric hospitals and patients being treated for emotional or behavioral disorders in general hospitals." If the reader stops reading after the phrase "This requirement applies only to psychiatric hospitals," he or she may come to the conclusion that the requirement is not applicable to his or her facility if it is not a psychiatric hospital.

If the person was to continue reading, the key phrase of "and patients being treated for emotional or behavioral disorders in general hospitals" nails the applicability to most general hospitals that operate an emergency room and typically have patients presenting with behavioral health disorders. This is the reason for using a team versus an individual to score. We continuously check ourselves for accuracy. The question on the table should be something similar to: "Do we as a general hospital ever treat psychiatric or behavioral conditions?" If you have psychiatrists on staff or are contracted with behavioral specialists for conducting assessments, you are treating psychiatric or behavioral conditions.

If you are unsure whether a category C EP is compliant and no existing data have been collected, consider collecting data from a few records (say, five or 10) to assess the EP. It doesn't take many to determine whether there is a problem. For your convenience, Figure 4.3 shows a simple data collection form that you can use for this task.

Internally Assessing Standards Compliance

Figure 4.3 ■ Data Collection Worksheet

Activity _____

Time frame or date _____

Data collected by _____

KEY: **Y** = indicator is met   **N** = indicator is not met   **N/A** = indicator not applicable

	Medical Record # →										Totals	
Indicators ↓											Yes	No

Document the Evidence of Compliance

Compliance determination may take you down many paths. Let's look at some of the common verbiage contained within EPs that should alert you to what is needed when assessing compliance.

LD.02.02.01 EP 1 requires the governing body to define, in writing, conflicts of interest involving leaders ... The words jumping off the page are *in writing* and *define*. An individual scoring this EP should search for a document addressing leadership conflict of interest. *Note:* This EP also is labeled with an icon consisting of a circle with a *D* in it; this icon indicates that either a document is required or documentation is required. Reading further into the EP provides the answer that a document is required.

MM.08.01.01 EP 1 addresses the need for the hospital to collect data on its medication management system. The collection of data could be initiated in multiple locations, but when this wording is found, begin your inquiries with personnel from the performance improvement department. If they are not accountable for the data collection, chances are they will be aware of where such data are being collected.

The terms *authoritative resources*, *evidence-based*, and *best practices* are used in various EPs. Here are a few examples:

- **NPSG.03.05.01 EP 4**, where authoritative resources are referenced for managing potential food and drug interactions for patients taking the medication warfarin
- **NPSG.07.03.01 EP 5**, which references compliance with evidence-based guidelines or best practices in regard to multidrug-resistant organisms
- **PC.02.01.11 EP 4**, which requires an evidence-based training program for resuscitative techniques

When such terms are used in an EP, the organization must have evidence that it has selected an entity that provides materials that are evidence-based, meaning they are backed up with research from the Centers for Disease Control and Prevention; or authoritative, as in standard-setting similar to the American College of Emergency Physicians; or best practices, as outlined in core measures for congestive heart failure.

> **Key Concept**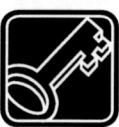
>
> Before the EP can be scored, the individual(s) responsible for the task must be consulted as to what material has been adopted. The entity, title, and year of publication should be documented as the evidence for compliance.

Assessment versus "Parking Lot" Issues

When we assemble a team of employees to tackle the tedious job of evaluating practices, particularly when it is aimed at assessing work processes, we sometimes get bogged down in all the problems and we can't move on to the task at hand, which is the assessment. It seems as though every policy we pull contains errors, changes from years ago were never updated in documents, personnel who originally authored a document are no longer employed, and the list goes on.

When it feels like your wheels are spinning, stop and reevaluate your mission. Can the EPs still be scored based on the requirements? If the answer is yes, note the other problematic issues identified on a flipchart, often referred to as the "parking lot," and stay focused on scoring. If the answer is no, record noncompliance and note that the steps to correction may need to include the identified issues. Be very careful that your team is not overcalling noncompliance because they are tangled in minutia and have lost focus of what the EP is requiring.

Categorize the Noncompliant Findings for Action

The internal assessment results are a snapshot in time of your organization's compliance. Once deficiencies are identified, organizations need to develop and implement action plans, measure progress, and monitor compliance with the goal of achieving improvements for the long term.

But before you move into action plans, it may help you to think of noncompliant standards by dividing them into the following three categories:

- **Easy fix:** A slight change in a document that doesn't require multiple committee approval or a minor change in practice involving only one patient care. Usually can be resolved in several days.

- **Moderate fix:** Involves document and practice changes in more than one patient care area. May take several weeks to research and obtain consensus. Education or training will be required, but not in a formalized setting; a newsletter, staff meetings, and so forth shall suffice.

- **Major fix:** Involves the medical staff as well as employees. Policy or procedure requires significant revisions to meet the EPs that lead to a noncompliant standard. Implementation must be structured, and in some areas, training to achieve competency may be warranted.

By categorizing the noncompliant standards, a fairly surprising number may be broken down into an easy fix where they can be promptly corrected even before there is a need to enter them into an action plan. Consider including the effect of noncompliance to patient safety and quality of care. When presenting the results of the internal assessment to leadership, the impact on patient safety and quality may influence their decision-making for allocating resources to correct the noncompliance.

Report the Initial Results to Key Stakeholders

When the results of a thorough internal assessment are tallied, teams often are surprised at the number of findings. Almost always, someone raises the question, "If we have this many noncompliant standards, how have we made it through our past surveys?" And you will already have the answer: Surveys do *not* assess each and every EP found in the applicable standard manual! This is why categorizing findings is important—so that people will not have "sticker shock" when they see the first aggregation of noncompliance numbers.

Do not be surprised if someone says, "This cannot be right! These numbers have to be wrong. Who did this? Do they know what they are doing?" Anyone who has been on the receiving end of these types of comments know that the integrity of the internal process will be in question; that is why we must be very careful to apply the recommended steps of performing an internal assessment previously described in this chapter.

> **Field Experience**
>
> Prepare the initial results as a summary by standards. Even though the scoring occurs at the EP level, there are just too many EPs to report their findings. Some organizations have listed the outcomes data by chapters, indicating the total number of standards, those scored compliant, and those scored noncompliant; then, after the noncompliant section, they list a breakdown by category. If you think this is too much detail for your organization, consider rolling the count into a simple number of noncompliant standards and the breakdown by categories. Keep the focus on moving toward continuous standards compliance and don't get waylaid by the count, especially if the number is larger than anticipated. If the work of the teams is undercut at this point, the organization will be hard-pressed to obtain staff members who are willing to work on the action plans.

Begin the Improvement Process

After conducting the internal assessment, you must address noncompliant standards. You can use any type of action plan, but it must be in writing and actively utilized to motivate staff members to continue to plug along until compliance is achieved. A simple table may serve as an action plan; a sample is displayed in Figure 4.4.

For each action step, enter a person's name in column two to be accountable for following the item to completion or communicating an existing roadblock. Do not list committees or departments as responsible parties, because such ambiguity results in no action. Use a "go to green approach": As the task is completed, highlight the task in green as a visual for team members to see their progress.

Project a completion date for each step. Consider utilizing the action plan as the agenda for the meeting that oversees continuous survey readiness. Energies should be focused on the noncompliant items and "getting to green."

Keep the actions moving and do not hesitate to address a roadblock at the appropriate level in the organization. In some situations, leadership may acknowledge noncompliance and place actions on hold due to budget restraints or a lack of resources. This should be noted on the action plan so that the team can move on to other issues and stop spinning their wheels.

Figure 4.4 ■ TJC Continuous Survey Readiness Action Plan

Chapter Team: Medication Management

Minimal Information (MM.1.10/EP2)	Person(s) to Address	Action Steps	Target Date	Status
Pregnancy and lactation is not consistently being collected on entry/admission. Info is not consistently being provided to the pharmacy.	Sara Jones Bob Smith Bob Smith Lynda Mart TBD	• Research whether data fields are available on assessment forms used in outpatient and inpatient patient care units. • Request revision of user defined fields within electronic nursing assessment used in outpatient surgery to include pregnancy and lactation • Work with IT for data transfer to pharmacy • Test system • Provide instructions to involved staff • Implement process • Review 30 records	12-3-08 12-29-08	11-13 Awaiting response from software company; called twice

Source: TJC Survey Coordinator's Handbook, Ninth Edition © 2007 HCPro, Inc.

Why Do Internal Assessments Sometimes Fail?

Limited resources to conduct an internal assessment

This may be more applicable in smaller hospitals for persons who already are accountable for several functions. It is impossible to be an expert in all fields, and the time factor may be too overwhelming for performing the internal assessment.

Staff reductions have left remaining staff members overwhelmed. A request to take on one more task may be met with much resistance. Leadership support will be needed to overcome this situation.

Failure to assess practice in addition to policies/procedures

Failure also occurs when an internal assessment is conducted in the meeting room without the input of those who perform the function. An assessment of the paper process looks great, but no one actually determines what is accruing in the day-to-day work setting. This method may have worked in older survey methods before tracer methodology was implemented, but not anymore. Observations of actual practice and interviews of active staff members will be concurrently assessed.

Easy fixes not prioritized; volume of corrections too daunting

It is not unusual to find practices that are in compliance, but the document that provides the structure for the process is outdated and differs in content. These problems are easy to fix, but often are not addressed. They become lumped in with all the other complex issues and forgotten. The survey occurs, these easy fixes are cited, and someone says, "I thought these were fixed!"

Underscoring results in a false sense of security

Do not be afraid to score an EP as noncompliant. Look at the document that describes the expected practice for category A EPs and compare the wording to the requirements. For category C EPs, seek data that have been collected. If such data do not exist, a quick collection of even 10 records/observations/interviews will provide you with information regarding whether the practice is in place. "Soft" scoring is a waste of time and might come back to bite you in an actual survey.

Failure to incorporate standards into routine operating processes

When we try to perform a task without understanding its rationale and the reasons for improving patient care and safety, the task is only temporary and will not become part of our habitual practices.

Tasks added onto routine operating processes require active thinking to perform the function. Our goal is to promote understanding and build habitual practice into an individual's "hard drive" so that the right thing is done first from understanding and then from habit.

An example is hand hygiene. Cleansing the hands before and after touching a patient should become so habitual that active thinking is no longer necessary. Once an individual understands the role of hand hygiene in preventing the occurrence of infections and the products are readily available, the act of hand hygiene becomes automatic.

The Joint Commission standards should be integrated with organizational policies and procedures to achieve continuous compliance. As noncompliant standards are corrected, try to work on enhancing an existing process instead of building something completely new. People are much more amenable to amending a practice than they are at starting over.

Sustaining Compliance

For individuals directly involved in coordinating accreditation activities, sustaining compliance presents many challenges. It is human nature to take a deep breath after completing the internal assessment and be glad it is over! Unfortunately, our work is never over if we are to achieve continuous compliance and cease the roller-coaster effect of slack off, intensify, slack off, intensify. To plan our strategies, we need to understand why some leaders are not on board with the concept of continuous compliance.

Historically, the fallback to a one-person method of preparation usually worked because the "old" survey method consisted of showcasing documents in organized manuals, arranging meetings with the surveyors, and attempting to restrict unit visits to the locations that were the most prepared. Today's approach, although more challenging, comprises observation and interviews to assess actual operations as the patient moves through the hospital system. To have a successful survey, hundreds of patient caregivers must be involved. Nothing is staged. It is the read deal on survey day.

Why are some leaders slow to buy into continuous readiness?

Many leaders who have experienced an unannounced survey actually agree that this approach is less disruptive to operations and better represents standards compliance. But we still have some leaders who are slow to change their thinking, and the following may be some of the reasons:

- Surveyor variation continues to exist, and leaders believe they can establish an on-site rapport that will persuade surveyors to look the other way or be more lenient when noncompliant standards are identified. The Joint Commission is continually working to strengthen surveyor skills and decrease surveyor/standards interpretation variation. It behooves leadership to promote actual standards compliance and not to count on surveyor disparity.

- Leaders know of organizations that have received multiple RFIs that were easily clarified away post-survey, so they believe it is an easy fix should their organization not comply. Unfortunately, such leaders knew only half of the story. Surveyor scoring errors were often the basis for "easy clarifications," or additional data collection yielded an RFI reversal. The bottom line is that the organization still needed to improve processes to avoid a repeat of the situation.

- Listservs and informal communication methods still advocate that there is a way to determine when you will be surveyed. CEOs hear this, and they think they still have time to ready the team at the last minute.

- Mock surveys may be conducted by an external entity, resulting in multiple findings of noncompliance. (I often refer to this as "Fayco Jayco" to encourage my clients to open up and learn from the assessment process.) The organization's subsequent Joint Commission survey does not yield the same findings of noncompliance, or perhaps not even the volume of RFIs. Leaders draw their own conclusion that they were "ready enough." We all need to remember that only a very small subset of standards and EPs are assessed by either Fayco Jayco or the real deal. The subset of standards may be totally different, and therefore not an exact comparison of readiness.

Conduct internal tracers

> **Field Experience**
>
> Conducting internal tracers seems to be the most efficient way to determine whether practices meet standards. Tracer activities can be very helpful in evaluating existing practices, but you can also use them to determine whether revised processes or newly implemented processes are actually in place and staff members are able to articulate the changes. Feedback from clients who have implemented a well-structured tracer process has provided testimonials of success. Included in the appendix of this book is a "Show Me" tracer developed by Janelle Holth and Jodi Sorum at Altru Health System in Grand Forks, ND. This innovative tool focuses on some of the most frequently cited standards and was designed to observe that actual compliance had been implemented.

Formulate a schedule of locations to be traced. Assign a team of two to conduct the tracer. Team up an individual from a noninpatient setting with an inpatient caregiver. And don't forget to include leadership. A CEO once told me that it made a much bigger difference to him to actually see a record with a missing history and physical than to hear about it from a medical record review summary report.

Provide feedback to individuals involved in the care of the patient who was traced. Both positive and negative feedback should be provided. It is a principle of adult learning that behaviors are more likely to change when an individual receives direct feedback. Figure 4.5 displays one method of "You've Been Traced."

Internally Assessing Standards Compliance

Figure 4.5 ■ You've Been Traced

[*Hospital Logo*]

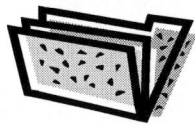 **You've been traced!**

Staff/Physician Name _____

Date _____

We believe it is important to provide individual feedback regarding employee and medical staff documentation and observed practices as assessed during patient tracer activity.

Tracer methodology evaluates patient care in the multiple settings where the patient was treated during their encounter.

❏ Great documentation! The tracer team identified the following exemplary patient care documentation:
_____
_____
_____

❏ Opportunities for improvement regarding your documentation were identified during this tracer:
_____
_____
_____

❏ Great practice observed!
_____
_____
_____

❏ Opportunities for improving practice:
_____
_____
_____

The Joint Commission Survey Coordinator's Handbook, 11th Edition

Integrate data collection efforts

Another mechanism that may streamline compliance activities is to integrate findings from the internal assessment, tracer activities, and applicable performance improvement data collection. Determine what data are needed to measure some of the most common category C EPs and collaborate with the performance improvement department before initiating further data collection efforts. Do not attempt to maintain one set of data for the Joint Commission survey and another for the performance improvement department.

Keep the action plan visible

Each department and discipline continues to have its own priorities, and they may or may not coincide with standards compliance. It's up to a hospital's leaders to establish organizational priorities and hold people accountable for working together to make improvements. One of the best ways to do this is to keep the action plan for continuous standards compliance on people's meeting agendas. If "go to green" is the ideal, consider color-coding those departments that are not making progress as red and deficiencies that are making slower than desired progress as yellow.

> **Success Story**
>
>
> One organization added a column to its action plan that listed the vice president who provided oversight to the individual assigned to the specified tasks. If progress was not occurring, the written inquiry was forwarded to the vice president along with the individual's name.

Be willing to try whatever it takes to keep leaders informed and knowledgeable of the organization's vulnerabilities so that there will be no surprises on the day the team arrives and announces, "We are from The Joint Commission, and we are here to perform your standards compliance survey."

In reality, an internal assessment is actually never complete. It is a dynamic process that is edited and updated as services, operations, and standards change. The more thorough an organization is in concurrently updating its internal assessment tool, the less it will have to scramble at the time of "touch points," introduced at the beginning of this chapter. Imagine a meeting of the core group who conducted the previous internal assessment where the meeting is simply an oversight of any changes entered concurrently during the past year. No additional EP reviews, no digging for documents, no updating of policies, and no last-minute educational sessions. When this occurs, congratulations; you will have achieved continuous compliance.

TEST YOUR KNOWLEDGE

1. True or false: The Joint Commission only allows the organization's designated software administrator to have access to the extranet site.

Answer: False. The individual designated as the extranet administrator is allowed to set up access parameters and pass codes for multiple individuals within the organization.

2. Which of the following are considered extensions of the standards manual by The Joint Commission?
- A. *Perspectives*
- B. FAQ responses
- C. Account executive inquiries
- D. Responses from the Standards Interpretation Group (SIG)

1. A and B
2. A and C
3. B and C
4. C and D

Answer: 1. Even though information from the account executive and SIG is helpful, The Joint Commission only recognizes items published in *Perspectives* and FAQ responses to be binding for surveyors to review against.

CHAPTER 5

Life Safety Code Compliance for the Nonengineer

The *Statement of Conditions* (LS.01.01.01)

The National Fire Protection Association (NFPA) writes codes for other agencies and authorities to adopt. It is important to understand that the NFPA does not enforce any of the codes that it writes. All of its codes are created by consensus, by committees made up of people who work with the codes on a daily basis. The NFPA 101 *Life Safety Code® (LSC)* is a code to protect lives from the harmful effects of fire, and this is accomplished by many different requirements. The *LSC* was originally written as a code that defines the appropriate components of exiting from a building in case of fire, which is still a large portion of the code. It has evolved to be a code that is comprehensive in all aspects of building safety, from the type of construction used to the requirements for fire detection and suppression.

The Joint Commission is one of the many authorities—among them the Centers for Medicare & Medicaid Services (CMS)—that has adopted the 2000 Edition of the *LSC* as the standard to use for protecting building occupants from fire. Although more recent editions of the *LSC* have been written since 2000, The Joint Commission and CMS are still using the 2000 Edition.

The *Statement of Conditions (SOC)* is a Joint Commission document that requires the hospital to assess the building for compliance with the *LSC*. This document is usually filled out by the facilities department and is now found in electronic form on the Joint Commission Connect secure Web site, replacing the older paper version of the *SOC*.

There are two parts to the *SOC*: the Basic Building Information (BBI) portion and the Plan for Improvement (PFI) portion. The hospital is required to enter basic information about the building in the

BBI portion for all healthcare occupancies (hospitals and ambulatory and long-term care facilities) as well as business occupancies (office buildings) that are used for exiting from a healthcare occupancy.

After the assessment for compliance with the *LSC* has been made and deficiencies have been identified, the hospital has multiple options involving those deficiencies:

- Repair/resolve the deficiencies right away

- If they cannot be resolved immediately but can be resolved within 45 days, enter them into the hospital's computerized maintenance management system for resolution

- If they cannot be resolved within 45 days of discovery, enter them in the PFI portion of the *SOC*

- Consider requesting an equivalency from The Joint Commission if an acceptable level of safety is present (if approved, the deficiency does not have to be resolved)

When entering information in the PFI portion, it is extremely important to have realistic projected start dates and projected completion dates. Once a Joint Commission surveyor has accepted the *SOC*, your organization cannot change these dates except through special written permission from The Joint Commission. Although you are automatically granted a six-month extension without having to ask for it, if your organization has exceeded the projected completion date by more than six months without an extension granted by The Joint Commission, you will be scored CON-04 and conditional accreditation will be revoked. Therefore, it is critically important to monitor projected completion dates on all PFIs to ensure that your organization is not past due.

Compliance tip

Ask to see the *SOC* for your organization and look for the projected completion dates of all the PFIs to validate that they are completed on time.

Required documentation

- Electronic *SOC*, or e-*SOC* filled out on the Joint Commission's secure extranet Web site

- The paper copy (if applicable) of the *SOC* from your last triannual survey for the surveyors to review the completion dates on the PFI list

- A letter or memo from your senior leadership that identifies and authorizes an individual (or vendor, if applicable) who is qualified to complete the *SOC* for your organization

Life Safety Code Compliance for the Nonengineer

Interim Life Safety Measures (LS.01.02.01)

The hospital is required to write a policy explaining what interim actions will be taken when a life safety feature is impaired due to construction, maintenance, or system failure. This is commonly referred to as the Interim Life Safety Measure (ILSM) policy. In this policy, you are required to list criteria for evaluating what actions will be taken, along with who will take those actions, when, and how, for specific life safety provisions that are identified in LS.01.02.01.

Every deficiency to a life safety feature must be assessed for interim measures according to your ILSM policy. As a result of this assessment, you determine what actions, if any, are appropriate to take to compensate for the deficiency. In addition to ILSM actions, you must notify the local fire department and initiate a fire watch whenever the fire alarm or sprinkler system is out of service for more than four hours in a 24-hour period in an occupied building. This notification must be documented and is best accomplished by sending the fire department a fax transmission.

Temporary systems used to compensate for impaired life safety systems must be tested/inspected once every month. If a fire watch is used due to an impaired system, it needs to be inspected once per month. You can accomplish this by conducting an audit of the record log for each fire watch inspection.

Compliance tip

Ask to see the ILSM assessments for each PFI on the *SOC*. By definition, a PFI is a life safety deficiency, and therefore it must be assessed for ILSMs.

Required documentation

- An ILSM policy

- Assessments of life safety deficiencies for ILSMs

- Notification of the local fire department when the fire alarm or sprinkler system is out of service for four or more hours in a 24-hour period

- Monthly tests/inspections of temporary systems used due to an impaired life safety feature

Chapter 5

Minimizing the Effects of Fire and Smoke (LS.02.01.10)

The *LSC* specifies certain types of construction for hospitals. The most common types are structural steel and brick or stone fascia. However, in some special situations, wood frame construction may be allowed. New construction must include automatic fire suppression systems (sprinklers), and some construction types require sprinklers in existing construction.

Fire-rated walls must reach from the floor to the slab above, through any interstitial spaces. Openings in fire-rated walls (doors) must be approved as fire-rated and have positive latching hardware, with a door-closing device. Doors may not have decorations or other coverings applied to their faces, with the exception of informational signs.

Heating, ventilation, and air-conditioning ductwork that penetrates two-hour fire resistance–rated walls, or vertical shaft walls of any fire rating, must have fire dampers inside the duct at the point where the duct penetrates the barrier. The fire damper must be fire-rated for at least one and a half hours. All pipes, wires, and conduits that penetrate fire-rated barriers must be sealed with fire-rated materials.

Safety tip

Ask to review your facilities department inspection records of all fire doors in the hospital, looking to ensure that all fire doors were actually inspected. Although inspection records are not required, they are an indication that this important feature of life safety is inspected and maintained.

Means of Egress (LS.02.01.20)

Doors must be unlocked in the direction of egress and swing in the direction of egress when the occupant capacity is 50 people or more. There are some exceptions to this requirement; the most common involves behavioral health units. You are permitted to lock the exit doors to keep your clients inside the unit, provided all staff members working in the unit have a key or device on their person to unlock the door.

Stairs and ramps in existing buildings must have hand rails on at least one side. Corridors in existing hospitals must be at least 4 feet wide. However, when renovating existing hospitals, you are not allowed to reduce the width of the corridor to that which is required for new construction. Corridors in new hospitals are required to be 8 feet wide, so corridors in existing hospitals must remain their current width or be modified to be at least 8 feet wide.

The maximum wall protrusion into the corridor is 3.5 inches, with the exception of items such as alcohol-gel hand rub dispensers and retractable wall-mounted computer desks. These items may protrude up to 6 inches into the corridor.

Corridors, exit access corridors, exit discharges, and exits must be free and clear of all obstructions, including unattended items in the path or egress. An unattended item is anything left in the corridor for 30 minutes or more that is not actively being used by anyone. A sure sign is anything plugged into a wall outlet in the corridor—it's a good bet that item is being stored there. The 30-minute window allows nursing staff members to temporarily stage items while rearranging a patient's room.

Exit doors are not allowed to be covered with any device that could obstruct them or confuse occupants as to their use. This means decorations, mirrors, draperies, and similar items are not permitted on these doors.

Suites are special designated areas that are considered one large room, with many other smaller rooms inside. Common examples of suites are intensive care units (ICU), emergency departments, operating rooms, and radiology departments. The beauty of a suite designation is that all hallways inside the suites are no longer exit access corridors, and therefore there is no minimum width requirement. Also, there are no restrictions to unattended items left in the hallway. Other advantages include:

- The interior walls of the suite are nonrated, and therefore maintenance and inspections are not required.

- Interior doors are not required, so if you have them, they are not required to positively latch. This is a great asset for suites with ICU patient rooms, as they frequently have sliding glass doors that do not latch.

However, there are certain requirements for suites that make it difficult for some areas to qualify:

- Suites for patient sleeping rooms are limited to no more than 5,000 square feet

- Suites for areas other than patient sleeping rooms are limited to 10,000 square feet

- Travel distance from the farthest point in the suite to an exit door of a suite for areas other than patient sleeping rooms is 100 feet when traversing one intervening room, and 50 feet when traversing two intervening rooms

- Travel distance from the farthest point in a suite to an exit door for areas serving patient sleeping rooms is limited to 100 feet

- All suites must be arranged so that no intervening room is a hazardous room

- Suites larger than 1,000 square feet that are used for patient sleeping rooms, and suites larger than 2,500 square feet that are used for something other than patient sleeping rooms, must have two or more exit doors that are remotely located from each other

- Doors to suites have to close and latch and must be rated the same as any other door in the corridor

The means of egress is required to be adequately illuminated. The means of egress is defined as all corridors, exit passageways, stairwells, exit discharge, and the path to the public way (outdoors). All points and angles must be illuminated to at least 2-foot candles, which is not very much light—about the light provided by two lit matches. The light fixtures must be arranged so that if one bulb burns out, the means of egress is still illuminated. This can be accomplished with multiple light fixtures or one light fixture with multiple bulbs.

Exit signs are required only when the path to the exit is not readily apparent. There is an old myth that surveyors perpetuated that required at least two exit signs be visible at all times and at all points in an exit access corridor. This is not true. If the path to an exit is readily apparent, such as the main entrance at the front of the hospital, an exit sign is not required.

Compliance tip

When you are making rounds and you see what appear to be unattended items in the corridor, ask your staff how long the items have been in the corridor without anyone using them. If they have been there for more than 30 minutes, that is an excellent opportunity to give a lesson about such objects.

During holiday periods, walk around and see whether your staff is placing decorations on exit doors or fire-rated doors. Inappropriate decorations are typically found on doors from Halloween through Valentine's Day.

Nothing in the *LSC* prevents a hospital from retroactively creating a suite in an area as long as it qualifies. In other words, this is not something that needs architectural design or Joint Commission approval. However, check with your local and state agencies to determine whether you need their approval before proceeding.

Ask to review your facilities department inspection records on the illumination of the means of egress, looking to ensure that all lights and lamp fixtures were actually inspected. Although inspection records are not required, they are an indication that this important feature of life safety is inspected and maintained.

Patient room doors in behavioral health units are permitted to be locked from the corridor side, provided there is a means to unlock and open the door with a single action from the inside. Hospitals sometimes like to lock vacant rooms to keep unauthorized individuals from entering. The doors must be able to be unlocked from the inside in case someone is accidentally locked in.

Protection from Hazards of Fire and Smoke (LS.02.01.30)

Vertical openings, such as stairwells, elevator shafts, ventilation shafts, communication stairs, ramps, light shafts, trash and linen chutes, and utility chases must be constructed to a one- or two-hour fire rating, depending on the height of the building.

Hazardous areas must be either contained with fire-rated construction, or protected with sprinklers, or both. Hazardous areas are defined as:

- Boiler rooms
- Laboratories
- Laundries larger than 100 square feet
- Flammable liquid storage rooms
- Flammable compressed gas storage rooms
- Maintenance repair shops
- Piped oxygen (or nitrous oxide) gas manifold supply rooms
- Paint shops

- Soiled linen rooms

- Storage rooms larger than 50 square feet containing combustibles

- Trash collection rooms

- Gift shops storing or displaying combustibles

In all applications, the entrance door to each of these rooms needs to have positive-latching hardware and a door-closing device.

Corridor walls have to extend from the floor to the slab above and be fire-rated and smoke-resistant if the smoke compartment is not fully protected with automatic sprinklers. If the smoke compartment is fully protected with automatic sprinklers, the corridor walls may terminate at the ceiling level as long as the ceiling limits the transfer of smoke. This means there are no requirements for fire-rated walls above the ceiling in the corridors protected with sprinklers.

Doors in corridors, such as doors to offices and patient rooms, are not required to have door closures but must have positive-latching hardware or a means to keep the door closed with a minimum of 5 lbs. of force. The latter is difficult to maintain and is not recommended. The following corridor doors are exempt from latching:

- Doors to toilet rooms

- Bathroom doors

- Shower room doors

- Sink closet doors

At least two smoke compartments are required on any story where more than 30 patients are housed. Smoke compartments are used as an area of refuge whenever there is a fire: Staff members relocate patients from one smoke compartment to another to escape the effects of a fire. Smoke compartment barriers are required to be fire-rated and the doors to smoke compartments are required to have closures, but they are not required to positively latch. Unlike corridor walls, smoke compartment barriers must extend from the floor all the way to the slab above, regardless of whether your compartment is protected with sprinklers.

Compliance tip

During rounds, take a look at your gift shop. It is likely that there are enough combustibles in the gift shop to make it qualify as a hazardous room. Examine the doors to the gift shop: Do they close and latch? Is there a door closure? When the door closes, does it resist the passage of smoke? Any "no" answer is a deficiency with the *LSC*.

As you perform rounds, be in the habit of tugging or pushing on corridor doors to make sure they actually close and latch. Report all doors that do not latch to your maintenance department.

During rounds, ask your staff where the closest smoke compartment barrier is located. It is critically important that they know exactly where the smoke compartment barriers are located so that they know where to evacuate their patients in the event of a fire. Hint: Not all cross-corridor doors that are held open with magnets are smoke compartment doors. If the smoke compartment doors are not obvious, ask your facilities department to mark them in some fashion (e.g., small signs, special color, etc.) so that everyone will recognize them as smoke compartment doors.

Fire Alarm Systems and Sprinkler Systems (LS.02.01.34 and LS.02.01.35)

Your hospital is required to have an approved operating fire alarm system. Although manual pull stations are required for healthcare occupancies, smoke detectors are not required everywhere. Certain requirements involving smoke detectors are dependent on many variables in your hospital. See the Environment of Care chapter for testing and maintenance requirements.

Your hospital may or may not be required to have sprinklers. New construction requires sprinklers, but existing construction does not. In addition, certain construction types require sprinklers regardless of whether the facility is considered new or existing. However, there are many advantages to a fully sprinklered hospital, including:

- Corridor wall construction
- Travel distance to exits
- Fire-rated construction for hazardous rooms
- Smoke dampers in smoke compartment barriers

You must maintain at least 18 inches of clearance from the sprinkler head to items stored on the top shelf or any other tall object. The exception to this rule applies to shelves that are tight up against the wall and are not directly underneath a sprinkler head.

Portable fire extinguishers are required throughout the hospital, in strategic locations, and the type and size must be matched to the potential fire. Figure 5.1 provides a chart to help you identify the requirements.

Fire extinguishers are required to be inspected monthly and annually. The monthly inspection can be accomplished by your own staff. Testing and inspection requirements for sprinkler systems and other fire suppression systems are found in the Environment of Care chapter.

Figure 5.1 ■ Requirements for Portable Fire Extinguishers

Hazard Classification	Hazard Occupancy	Minimum Fire Extinguisher Rating	Travel Distance
Class A	Low	2-A	75 ft.
Class A	Moderate	2-A	75 ft.
Class A	High	4-A	75 ft.
Class B	Low	5-B	30 ft.
Class B	Low	10-B	50 ft.
Class B	Moderate	10-B	30 ft.
Class B	Moderate	20-B	50 ft.
Class B	Moderate	40-B	30 ft.
Class B	High	80-B	50 ft.
Class C	A Class C fire is started by an electrical means, but the fire itself is either a Class A or a Class B fire. Therefore, the travel distance and the size and type of extinguisher must be sized and located on the basis of the anticipated Class A or Class B hazard.		
Class K	A Class K extinguisher must be provided where hazards exist involving combustible cooking oils or fat.		30 ft.

Life Safety Code Compliance for the Nonengineer

Compliance tip

Ask to review your facilities department vendor inspection records on the fire alarm system and the sprinkler system in your organization. Take time to look specifically for any recommendations by the vendor to repair deficient devices discovered during the inspection. If you find any such notations, ask the facilities department for follow-up documentation that the devices were actually repaired or replaced.

Always support efforts by your organization to install sprinklers in places where they are not already installed. The added benefit for patient safety and the reduced expense in time and resources will far outweigh all up-front costs.

Take a tape measure with you during rounds, and check for the proper 18-inch clearance underneath sprinkler heads.

Take a look at fire extinguishers during rounds. They must be inspected once per month, but The Joint Commission says it can be anytime during the calendar month, not exactly 30 days, between inspections.

Building Services and Operating Features (LS.02.01.50 and LS.02.01.70)

Trash chutes must discharge directly into a holding room, and the holding room is not allowed to be used for any other purpose, such as storage.

Sprinklers are required inside all trash and linen chutes. A sprinkler head is required at the top and at the bottom and on every other floor in between.

The inlet doors to trash and linen chutes are required to be fire-rated and must have positive latching and a device to close the door. Access to the chute inlet door is required to be through a separate room, which is also required to be protected at the same fire rating as the chute enclosure.

Combustible decorations are not permitted in hospitals. There is no *LSC* requirement that decorations must be listed or approved by an independent testing laboratory, but they are not allowed to be combustible.

Soiled linen and trash containers larger than 32 gallons must be kept in a room designated as a hazardous room. Containers used to collect paper waiting to be shredded are considered trash containers for the purpose of this requirement.

Portable space heaters are not permitted in smoke compartments that contain patient sleeping or treatment areas. Portable space heaters with elements that exceed 212°F are not permitted.

Compliance tip

Check containers used to collect documents waiting to be shredded. If the container is larger than 32 gallons (the capacity of the container should be stamped on the top or bottom), ask your shredding vendor to replace it with containers smaller than 32 gallons.

Typically, oil-filled portable space heaters are the only type that meets the *LSC* requirement for heating elements that do not exceed 212°F.

In Conclusion

Compliance with the *LSC* is not a secret society where you need a special decoder ring or a fraternity handshake to figure it out. Like most codes and standards, it is based on common sense, practicality, and staff education.

The common sense part is just doing the right thing: We keep our corridors free from clutter because it is in the best interests for the safety of our patients. When a life safety feature is impaired, we compensate for it by implementing interim measures.

Suites of rooms are practical for an ICU. In a suite, the patient's room doesn't even need a door, let alone a latching door. And emergency response equipment is allowed to be left unattended in the hallway, just waiting to be used.

Compliance with the *LSC* is mostly a matter of educating staff members about certain requirements. Staff members need to know why it is important not to wedge open a door to a soiled utility room, because more fires begin in a utility room in a hospital than anywhere else. Sometimes it is helpful for people to know *why* before they can *do*. Life safety is just patient safety in the environment.

Note: See this book's online appendix for information regarding humidity and temperature monitoring in the operating room. A sample policy is provided, as well as additional information by *LSC* expert Brad Keyes.

Chapter 5

TEST YOUR KNOWLEDGE

1. True or false: CMS and The Joint Commission utilize the most recent publication of the *Life Safety Code* from the National Fire Protection Agency to evaluate hospitals.

Answer: False. They utilize the 2000 Edition even though updates have been published.

2. The Basic Building Information (BBI) portion of the *SOC* includes building information from which of the following settings?

    A. Long-term care
    B. Ambulatory care
    C. Business occupancies
    D. Hospital

    1. A, B, C
    2. B, C, D
    3. A, B, D
    4. All of the above

Answer: 4. All types of care settings are included in the organization's BBI.

3. Which of the following statements regarding life safety are true?

    A. Holiday decorations are temporarily permitted to be hung on fire doors as long as the decoration is made of a fire-retardant material
    B. Drop down–style computer desks may be used in hospital corridors but may not protrude any further than 6 inches
    C. Medical equipment may be in a patient care egress corridor on a temporary basis, which is defined as no longer than 30 minutes
    D. Exit doors to stairwells may be locked to prevent patient elopement as long as a key is readily available on the unit for quick unlocking

    1. A and C
    2. B and D
    3. B and C
    4. A and D

Answer: 3. At no time may any decorations be placed on fire doors. Also, when doors are locked on patient care units, all staff members must have a key on their person in the event of an emergency situation.

CHAPTER 6

The National Patient Safety Goals

Yes! No additions for 2010! Final revisions to the National Patient Safety Goals (NPSG) were posted to the Joint Commission Web site as a prepublished version on September 25, 2009. Since the inception of NPSGs in 2003, a record number of seven goals or portions of goal requirements were transferred into the chapter standards and the number of remaining goals has dropped to six (with a total of 14 standards), plus the Universal Protocol™ with its three standards.

While revising the NPSGs, language was clarified and some of the elements of performance (EP) were streamlined. It appears that the same type of scrutiny applied to the program standards in the Standards Improvement Initiative was used with the goal requirements. At first blush, the revisions appear to provide enhanced clarity of expectations. Except for the deleted requirements that were effective immediately, all other revisions are effective January 1, 2010.

For individuals who have memorized NPSG numbers or simply want a quick summary, Figure 6.1 shows a snapshot of the goals that remain.

At the time of this writing, Goal #8, Medication reconciliation, with four standards, is not in effect. Medication reconciliation continues to be evaluated and the language refined; it will not be scored until further notification from The Joint Commission sometime in the spring of 2010.

Figure 6.1 — Hospital NPSG 2010 Retained

Goal 1	Patient identification	• Two identifiers • Label specimen containers • Transfusion identification
Goal 2	Effective communication	• Critical results definition, reporting, timeline • Evaluate timeliness
Goal 3	Medication Safety	• Secondary labeling of containers • Anticoagulation therapy management
Goal 7	Infection prevention	• Hand hygiene compliance • MDRO management • Central line infection prevention • Surgical site infection prevention
Goal 8 (On hold)	Medication reconciliation	• Home medication list • Inpatient medication reconciliation • Discharge medication list provided • Outpatient medication reconciliation
Goal 15	Suicide risk	• Immediate safety • Prevention information to patient and family
Universal Protocol	Procedural safety	• Pre-procedure verification • Mark the site • Perform a time out

Moved NPSGs

As in previous years, the Joint Commission experts agree that the continued practice to improve patient safety is warranted, but some of the goals have had sufficient exposure to be moved into a chapter of the standards manual. Some of you will recall that this happened with concentrated electrolytes and the alarms on pumps and other medical equipment. Figure 6.2 provides another quick snapshot of where the NPSGs were relocated when they were moved into the chapter standards.

Figure 6.2 ■ Hospital NPSG 2010 Moved as of October 29, 2009

Goal 2	Read back of verbal orders	• New standard: PC.02.01.03 EP 20
	Do not use abbreviations	• Existing standard: IM.02.02.01 EPs 2 and 3 (managing health information)
	Handoff communication	• Existing standard: PC.02.02.02 EP 2 (coordinate patient's care)
Goal 3	Look-alike-sound-alike medications	• New standard: MM.01.02.01 EPs 1 - 3
Goal 9	Reduce harm from patient falls	• New standard: PC.01.02.08 EP 1 and 2 • Existing standard: HR.01.05.03 EP 8 (education and training) • Existing standard: PC.02.03.01 EP 10 (patient education) • Existing standard: PI.01.01.01 EP 38 (data collection)
Goal 13	Patient and family involvement	• Existing standard: PC.02.03.01 EP 27 (patient education) • Existing standard: IC.01.05.01 EP 7 (infection control plan) • Existing standard: IC.02.01.01 EP 7 (implementation of infection control plan)
Goal 16	Response to changes in patient's condition	• New standard: PC.02.01.19 EPs 1-4 • Existing standard: HR.01.05.03 EP 13 (education and training) • Existing standard: PI.01.01.01 EP 39 (data collection)

Key Concept

NPSGs that have moved to the standards have not disappeared; they are merely out of the spotlight of being goals. The expectation of implementation still exists. The exact verbiage of the moved EPs will not be known until The Joint Commission releases its updates to the standards manual.

Deleted NPSGs

Effective immediately following the publication of the October issue of *Perspectives,* surveyors were to discontinue scoring any NPSG requirement that had been deleted. Most of you cheered this because one of the most confusing and troublesome requirements was critical tests. As you may recall, critical tests were to be defined, data were to be collected to measure the timeliness of performing the tests, and the results were to be reported to the provider and action was to be taken to improve. You can rest assured that critical tests are now gone. If you conquered critical tests and found value in determining how quickly your organization could turn around a test deemed critical, there is no reason you have to cease evaluating. This should be an organizational decision. Such data collection is productive and improves response when patients with such diagnoses as impending cerebral vascular accident and acute myocardial infarction are cared for in the emergency department. It should also be noted that some disease-specific certifications have indicators that very closely resemble critical tests.

Another significant change for organizations that have achieved disease-specific certification is that only Joint Commission–accredited organizations may apply for the certification, so the set of NPSGs specific to the certification program has been eliminated. NPSGs as applicable to the disease-specific certification will be applicable and scored appropriately.

A Closer Look at Some of the Revisions for 2010

NPSG.02.03.01, Critical results

Take a careful look at your existing policy and procedure to determine that the individuals who report and the individuals they report to are clearly stated. A critical result may be identified for inpatients and outpatients, so ensure that follow-up for outpatients, especially after hours, has been defined.

Include all the diagnostic areas where critical results may be identified. Often, EKGs are performed on a routine basis and the computerized readout lists the results as abnormal but unverified. What is the responsibility of the technician in reporting these findings to the caregiver? Should certain computer readings be promptly called to the attention of a practitioner who is privileged to interpret EKGs so that a verified interpretation can be obtained?

> **Field Experience**
>
> Repeatedly during surgical tracers, a computerized reading of EKGs documents abnormal findings, sometimes indicative of an acute myocardial infarction, and the test has not been formally interpreted. On the preoperative checklist, EKG is checked off because it is on the record, not because it has been read. When asked, surgical staff members state that the anesthesia provider has "reviewed" the results. This is sometimes correct as there is a note relating the computerized results, but most anesthesia providers are not privileged to interpret 12 lead EKG results. Their expertise is in concurrent cardiac monitoring and recognition of abnormal tracings. For this reason, it is imperative that the definition of a critical result take into consideration preliminary computer readings so that acccurate interpretations can be sought for the sake of patient care and safety.

NPSG.03.04.01, Labeling of medication and solution secondary containers

If you consider the term *amount* to be synonymous with *quantity*, only two new items are now required to be included on labels:

- Preparation date

- Diluent and volume (if not apparent from the container)

It seems appropriate that the date of preparation would be noted on the container, especially for situations in which a nurse prepares a batch of heparin flushes for her daily hemodialysis patients that will be used over the course of her shift. Should any be inadvertently retained, the date would alert the next handler that disposal of the syringe is warranted. Some locations spike IV solution bags with tubing to increase the efficiency of IV insertions by estimating their need for the day. In this situation,

> **Key Concept**
>
> With the revision of this goal, an opportunity exists for your organization to promptly define what is considered a "short procedure" as the expiration date and time are not required for such procedures. Perhaps it would be based on a time frame of less than X hours, or it would be setting-specific—for instance, defining procedures performed in the interventional radiology department as "short." Don't create an entirely new policy; instead, retrieve your existing policy that addresses labeling of secondary medication and solution containers and make an addition under a specified heading.

In regard to the diluent, this goal is also applicable to solutions that frequently are mixed with another agent. Rarely do we see that agent listed on the label. Consider it similar to when a pharmacist prepares an admixture: The amounts of all ingredients are listed on the label. For solutions and medications that are consistently diluted, this may be the time to perform an inventory and arrange for preprinted labels to be prepared. Focus on the fact that the next person may not have a clue what is inside the container or syringe. The requirement for the labels to be both verbally and visually verified when the individual administering the medication or solution is not the person who prepared it remains a component of the goal. In the time it takes to argue the necessity of labeling, the labeling could have been done.

NPSG.03.05.01, Anticoagulation therapy

Dietary services no longer need to be notified of all patients receiving warfarin as a component of the food and drug interaction program. The use of "authoritative resources" is now allowed, which in most patient care practices will support what dietitians have been advocating: that the medication should be adjusted to the patient's usual diet. In addition, the volume of vitamin K–rich foods would need to be excessive to actually impact the effects of warfarin.

NPSG.07.01.01, Hand hygiene

The EPs for this goal have been changed from category C to category A. Before you panic and interpret that hand hygiene must be at 100% or you will receive a Requirement for Improvement (RFI), let's dissect the verbiage in the three EPs.

EP 1 requires that a program encompassing either the Centers for Disease Control and Prevention or the World Health Organization guidelines be *implemented*. Is there a hospital in the United States that has not implemented a hand hygiene program? I doubt it. So that EP is met.

EP 2 requires goals to be set for improving compliance. You may be asking whether this is similar to the goals we set following our infection control risk analysis. It is; so set a realistic goal based on your organization's current compliance rate, stretching for improvement. What is realistic? Who knows, but no one spells out the specifics for other performance improvement initiatives, so why should there be one for this goal? By analyzing your existing data, you might decide to set different goals for select areas. For example, suppose your post-anesthesia care unit is struggling with hand hygiene between patients because dispensers are at the head of the bed and curtained dividers prevent them from being placed at the exit point of the patient's bedside. The measurements of compliance have averaged 68% for the first three quarters of 2009. It is unrealistic to think that they will reach 100%, but could they push for a 10% increase by involving staff members in developing innovative interventions?

Key Concept

Incorporate the requirement of setting goals and improving compliance into your infection control risk assessment and strategies for improvement. Analysis of noncompliance will be critical to demonstrate that interventions correlate with the real causes of hand hygiene noncompliance. Here is where a Pareto chart could be helpful. A Pareto chart is a bar graph that presents data in descending order of importance. In this case, a Pareto chart could be used to show why noncompliance to hand hygiene guidelines is occurring and why (e.g., lack of knowledge, emergency response, product unavailable, etc.). Typically, the bars that make up 80% of the noncompliance will be the focus for improvement strategies. (An example Pareto chart has been included with the online materials at *www.hcpro.com/downloads/8088.*)

NPSG.07.03.01, NPSG.07.04.01, NPSG.07.05.01, Infection prevention

EP 3 requires improved compliance based on the goals your organization has established. If improvements are made, this EP will be scored compliant. Is 1% enough? Well, if you are at 93% and you increase by another 1%, I would say yes. You are pushing the group toward 100% compliance, and the going gets rough for achieving those last few percentage points (just as in weight loss, where the last few pounds are the toughest to lose). But if the organization or department was 68% noncompliant in the preceding example and moved to 69%, that is an insignificant improvement and I would expect the score to be noncompliance.

The three infection prevention NPSGs will be discussed together. Even though the topics are different, the approach to expectations and compliance is the same.

- NPSG.07.03.01, Implement evidenced-based practices for multidrug-resistant organisms
- NPSG.07.04.01, Preventing central line–associated bloodstream infections
- NPSG.07.05.01, Preventing surgical site infections

While the NPSGs were being revised, the timelines for implementation were removed. Regardless, time was drawing close for each organization to be on target for full implementation by January 1, 2010. If I were conducting a mock survey of these three goals, my questions might be the following:

1. What evidence-based guidelines did your organization select to guide you through compliance with the required EPs? Your answer should be the Centers for Disease Control and Prevention, the Institute for Healthcare Improvement, the Compendium of Strategies to Prevent Healthcare Associated Infections, and similar agencies.

2. Can you show me the results of your risk assessment?

3. How did you educate your physicians and caregivers on the requirements?

4. What methods were utilized to implement the policies and procedures?

5. What types of educational materials were prepared for patients or their families?

6. Where in the medical record is patient and family education documented?

7. What are the results of your process measures?

8. What are the results of your outcome measures?

9. Which key stakeholders are receiving reports of the measurements?

10. Based on your assessment of the effectiveness of the program, what improvement activities are being implemented, if applicable?

The sources suggested in question 1 are the most commonly utilized, but I am sure there are others. See the appendix for a listing of Web sites where you can find these documents and other resources.

NPSG.15.01.01, Decreasing suicide risks

Despite all the emphasis on this goal and the release of the Sentinel Event Alert in 1998, 100+ suicides were reported to The Joint Commission in 2008. Keep in mind that these are the *reported* suicides, and we know that many hospitals are not willing to report sentinel events.

To comply with EP 1, evidence of a risk assessment of the environment and specific patient characteristics must exist. The identification of risks should be minimized in settings where a patient's immediate safety needs are a priority. Naturally, behavioral health units are at the top of the list, but do not forget your emergency departments and intensive care units (ICU).

Field Experience

Some emergency departments continue to care for emotionally impaired patients in a room that contains equipment and environmental hazards that place the patient at increased risk for suicide. It is impossible to create a "safe room" by simply rolling out equipment that contains cords, IV tubing, sharps, and so forth. Work with your facilities staff and an expert in managing behavioral health patients at risk for harming themselves or others to perform a risk assessment.

Universal Protocol

Within the introduction of this goal, a wording change has occurred that may be problematic until clarification is published. Universal Protocol has historically been applied to all surgical and nonsurgical invasive procedures that "exposed the patients to more than minimal risk." Universal Protocol still states all surgical and nonsurgical invasive procedures, but adds the phrase "procedures that place the patient at the most risk include those that involve general anesthesia or deep sedation."

In addition, the phrase "a standardized list to verify availability" has replaced the term *checklist*. Plus, a note has been added to further clarify that an individual list for each patient need not be documented in the record, but instead, a tool such as a laminated worksheet can be used to ensure that the minimum items are ready or available for the procedure.

> **Key Concept**
>
>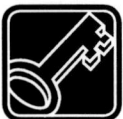
>
> Some adjustments have been made defining who may mark a surgical site, but the responsibility still remains with a provider who is privileged to perform the procedure and who will be present during the procedure if not actually performing the procedure. Qualified individuals such as residents, nurse practitioners, and physician assistants may, in "limited circumstances," be permitted to mark a surgical site. My recommendation is to sit tight and see how that rolls out in a FAQ on the Joint Commission's Web site. For organizations that struggled to have the physician perfoming the procedure held accountable for site marking, we do not want to go backward. Within the rationale of UP.01.02.01, The Joint Commission stated that there is no evidence that patient safety is affected by the person marking the site.

A little more latitude exists for defining alternative processes for patients who refuse site marking or when it is impractical. Examples of alterntives were not provided.

A change in the 2009 standards that added "conducting a timeout before anesthesia" was removed for 2010. This is good news, as the listing of multiple items to be included in a timeout is reduced back to the correct patient, correct site, and correct procedure. The expectation that team members will actively communicate has been moved from the EPs and is included in the rationale of UP.01.03.01. We will need to watch how this plays out in actual surveys. Only EPs are scored, so absence of verbalization should not result in a finding.

Old favorites still present problems

If we look at the statistics The Joint Commission published in the July 2009 issue of *Perspectives*, the following percentages of hospitals received RFIs for the listed NPSGs during 2008 surveys:

- Medication reconciliation: 19%
- Universal Protocol: 21%
- Labeling secondary containers: 25%
- Critical tests/critical values: 37%

These numbers tell us that we are still struggling to integrate NPSGs into our daily work routine following the natural course of processes ingrained within our work styles.

During consulting engagements, we often identify NPSG noncompliance practices. Many times it is the organization's own policy that unnecessarily raises the bar to an expectation that staff members cannot meet. For that reason, I recommend that you draft your policies using the word *require* to meet the minimal EPs, but strive for excellence by using the word *recommend* when stating goals that you would like staff members to reach. The Joint Commission will score practices against the defined EPs unless it discovers that your organization has a stricter policy, and therefore your policy trumps the EPs. When this happens, and it happens often during a survey, your organization will be scored against your own policy.

Field Experience

One of the most common findings is a policy addressing the time period for calling critical results to physicians. I have seen policies with such unrealistic goals: five minutes, for example. Think about that. In a busy ICU, you barely have time to hang up the phone, locate the physician's number, and dial the phone in five minutes! If the result is documented as six minutes, you are now noncompliant with your own hospital policy. And incidentally, this EP remains a category A EP (NPSG.02.03.01 EP 2), so that one-minute delay would be counted as a variance to the policy. (Recall that it takes only one finding to deem a category A EP noncompliant.) This scenario is just plain ridiculous, so don't paint yourself into a corner with over-restrictive policies. Knowing that the accreditation specialist has very little control over policy development, consider copying this section and sending it to all people involved in policy development.

Prudence or Wisdom: Can Your Policies Pass Muster?

WendySue Woods, RN, MHSA, CSHA, senior consultant with The Greeley Company, a division of HCPro, Inc., in Marblehead, MA.

In 1751, Dr. Thomas Bond and Benjamin Franklin founded the first hospital of the 13 colonies. At that time, Philadelphia was the fastest growing city, boasting a population in 1730 of 11,500 that grew to 15,000 in 1750. The mission of Pennsylvania Hospital, as it was then known, was "to care for the sick, the poor, and the insane who were wandering the streets of Philadelphia."

Patients were expected to follow strict rules and policies. They had to comply exactly with orders given by physicians and nurses. Talking was not allowed on the wards when the physicians were present. Patients could not be in their beds unless they were in bedclothes—no street clothes were allowed. There was to be no profane language, gambling, or spitting on the floors. The rule I like the best states that if you were able, you were expected to help the nurse with her duties. Imagine updating those policies to match practice today!

Don't Just Go through the Motions

Organizations have developed processes to ensure that policies are reviewed and revised as appropriate. This practice can vary a great deal from one organization to another. Many organizations divide their policies and they are reviewed and revised, often by people who do not have firsthand knowledge of the processes. Others may choose to accomplish this by committee, which results in policies being revised without the input of those who must comply with the policies.

Approximately 5% of the Joint Commission elements of performance (EP) are frequently cited. These are the Joint Commission EPs and the Centers for Medicare & Medicaid Services (CMS) requirements that seem to have the greatest impact on an organization's ability to consistently deliver quality and safe care. Consistency is the key, and this can be driven by a successful policy and procedure review process.

"Tag," You're It

When developing or revising a policy, "tag" that policy with the corresponding Joint Commission standard and EP as well as creating a link to the CMS *Conditions of Participation* "A" tag. Once you have this set up as a system, it will be easy to find the policy or policies and make the necessary changes as requirements and regulations are updated or changed.

Prudence or Wisdom: Can Your Policies Pass Muster? (Cont.)

Practice = Policy

During the revision or review process, take the policy to the bedside. Talk with the staff about the requirements and the methods they are currently using. Identify shortcuts that staff members have developed. Sometimes these are reasonable and still maintain compliance. Other times, these shortcuts can lead to missed steps, resulting in noncompliance. Take the time to talk with the staff to understand why the shortcuts or "workarounds" were implemented and help to keep the process sensible to the end user. This will ensure compliance and consistency. Practice will match policy.

Keep It Simple

Policies that are created from textbooks or in isolation often can create unreasonable expectations for end users. Implementation of the policy when put into practice and then placed under scrutiny can result in noncompliance because the steps did not make sense, and therefore they were not followed. Keep the process simple. Review the minimum expectations and align the policy accordingly. Just because something sounds good on paper does not mean it can be easily and consistently accomplished.

Take It for a Test Drive

Once a policy has been developed or reviewed and revised, kick the tires—take it for a spin. Think about what it would have been like to test the policy of "no talking when the physician is on the ward." How could the patient communicate his or her needs? How would the nurse have discussed the patient's condition and response to treatments? See whether the steps that have been outlined in the policy make sense to the staff members who will need to ensure implementation. Only then is the policy ready for a stamp of approval.

Educate and Assess

Once the policy has been developed, reviewed, or revised and you have taken it for a test drive, your work is not over. Ensure that staff members are educated or reeducated on the policy and any changes or nuances that need to be discussed. This piece of paper is only as good as the end user's ability to consistently comply with the requirements and demonstrate competence.

Chapter 6

> **Prudence or Wisdom: Can Your Policies Pass Muster? (Cont.)**
>
> **The Guidelines Today**
>
> If you were one of the excited lucky ones setting up the first hospital in the United States, you would have been writing the rules from scratch. That groundwork has long been established, but there are guidelines that can serve as valuable resources. The *2009 Comprehensive Accreditation Manual for Hospitals (CAMH): The Official Handbook* contains a chapter titled "Required Written Documentation." This chapter provides a list of all of the Joint Commission EPs requiring written documentation for hospitals. Not all of the items listed require policies—many are references to logs, licenses, annual reports, and so forth—but this is an excellent starting point for the prioritization process.
>
> Regardless of how your organization manages the process of developing, reviewing, and revising policies, invest the time to evaluate it to ensure that it can pass muster. Your process should give you the confidence that your patients are being consistently provided quality and safe care.

Use of two patient identifiers

There are two situations in which this is still tripping us up:

- During the delivery of therapeutic dietary trays
- Prior to transporting patients from patient care units

The delivery of patient trays has been a longstanding task of the food services department. Typically, a little tent with the patient's room number and name was on the corner of the tray. With the inability to use the room number as a patient identifier, another mechanism has to be implemented. If your organization is using patient-completed menus, consider tagging each meal section with a patient sticker that contains two patient identifiers. When that portion of the menu is placed back on the tray, the individual delivering the tray has a reminder in place to trigger the use of two identifiers.

> **Key Concept**
>
>  Test the practice during tracers by interviewing individuals in the process of passing trays. If you are using volunteers for this task, ensure that they have had adequate training to comply with this requirement.

Transporters tend to know the room number of the patient and the reason they have been asked to transport the patient, but beyond that they frequently arrive to the unit empty-handed. The following Field Experience sidebar provides a case in point.

> **Field Experience**
>
>
>
> Sometimes hospitals have multiple patients with the same name, particularly when the names are common to the hospital's geographical location and the culture of the population. A near miss occurred in a small hospital in Texas where the surgery transporter arrived at the inpatient desk to escort "Mr. Gonzalez" to the operating room. The conversation went something like this:
>
> > Transporter: "I'm here to pick up Mr. Gonzales in 302."
> > Nurse: "What's his first name?"
> > Transporter: "Juan."
> > Nurse: "Yes, he's in 302 and he's ready."
>
> In Preop Holding:
>
> > Nurse: "This is not the correct patient; he doesn't have a broken leg."
> > Transporter after checking the surgery schedule: "Oh, there is another Juan Gonzales in 516; he must be the right one."
>
> Transporters should always arrive to the unit with a requisition, schedule, face sheet, or some sort of document that includes two patient identifiers. Utilizing the document, the transporter should be educated to use the patient's arm band to compare the two identifiers on the patient's ID band to the document before transporting the patient. The patient care staff in attendance should not allow this requirement to be circumvented.

Labeling of secondary containers

Movement of medication into a syringe is to be a continuous process, with labeling and "drawing up" performed by one person. You may select your syringe, label it, and promptly draw up the medication, *or* you may select your syringe, draw up your medication, and immediately label it. That is the only variation allowed. If you choose not to label the syringe, you must immediately administer the medication. That syringe may not leave your hand and you can hold only the one syringe. If you require two syringes for the same patient, even if you go directly to the patient's room, each syringe must be labeled.

If you wish to avoid labeling, and instead prepare medications and solutions at the time of use, it is likely that you can vary your process and still be compliant with this safety goal. For example, take both the vial of medication and the syringe to the patient's bedside and do not prepare the medication until you are ready to administer it. If you need to examine the IV site or check the patient's vital signs, this is not a problem, as the medication has not yet been transferred to a secondary container.

Survey Emphasis on NPSGs

Regardless of the subject, the implementation of NPSGs is carefully scrutinized during individual patient and system tracer activities. Many of the goals are assessed through practice observation and cannot be measured through chart abstraction. That means your internal tracers should focus on the NPSGs that may be warranted to assist you in measuring compliance with these goals.

It is very important to periodically review the FAQs on the Joint Commission's Web site, as the answers may include additional interpretive information as well as compliance expectations that may be stated in a different way that provides clarity to the reader. Some of the FAQs are generated from actual questions submitted by staff members from accredited organizations. Accreditation specialists usually find the FAQs very helpful in applying some of the NPSGs to your facility's special circumstances. Remember, the FAQs are binding as if they were published components of the standards manual, so review them carefully.

Make it a habit
Many of the NPSGs are changes in practice that caregivers need to build and post to their own internal "hard drives" so that they become automatic safe practices. Staff members will know when that happens; for instance, when they reach for the hand sanitizer as automatically as they reach for the door knob to exit a room.

Patient safety is something that an individual must believe in and participate in to keep healthcare practices safe. As the accreditation specialist, you can assist in the process by introducing the safety behind the practice and pointing out the dangerous outcomes that have occurred when people stray from the safe practice in your own organization. Remember, The Joint Commission didn't create these goals to watch us pull our hair out. They are the result of patient deaths, injuries, and devastating outcomes, and we have a responsibility to ensure that these occurrences do not happen in our institutions. Provide staff members with the rationale behind the goals and ask for their assistance in rolling them out. And remind them that there will be a time when they, someone in their family, or their friend will be a patient. Let's start making it safer now.

TEST YOUR KNOWLEDGE

1. True or false: Revisions in the anticoagulation NPSG eliminate the requirement to notify dietary of all patients receiving warfarin.

Answer: True. Reference is made to utilizing authoritative resources to manage potential food and drug interactions. Dietitians continually expressed their concerns that a patient's diet would need to be greatly increased in greens and other foods rich in vitamin K to impact the effects of warfarin.

2. Which of the following are acceptable practices when transferring medications or solutions from their original container?
   A. Betadine poured into a cup need not be labeled on a sterile field set up for suturing as it is readily recognizable due to its dark brown coloring
   B. In the medication room, a nurse prepares an injection of fentanyl and carries the unlabeled syringe to the patient to administer the medication
   C. A half-strength solution of peroxide and normal saline is prepared by a nurse; the container is labeled "Oral rinse" along with the patient's two identifiers
   D. A syringe labeled with the name and strength of the medication and the preparation date is lying on the bedside stand in a patient's room as the patient has frequent pain

   1. All of the above
   2. None of the above
   3. B only
   4. A and B

Answer: 3. It is acceptable to prepare a medication and administer the medication. The medication must remain with the preparer and be promptly administered. The remaining answers are incorrect because the color of a well-known solution does not substitute for labeling; new for 2010, the diluent and the solution must be included on the label; and a syringe prepared by another person must be visually and verbally verified before it is administered.

CHAPTER 7

Ready, Set, Survey: Methods for Preparing for and Managing Your Survey

When we think about on-site surveys, the first thing that comes to mind is the fact that they are truly unannounced. We're nervous about when the surveyors will arrive, whether we will be ready for the scrutiny, and how well we will do with tracer activities. The change to unannounced arrivals definitely was significant in the survey process and can leave organizations vulnerable if they do not plan, prepare, and then prepare some more, as this is The Joint Commission's method for assessing whether an entity has taken continuous standards compliance to heart.

It appears that some folks are still grieving over their inability to set the dates, schedule the interviews, reserve the rooms, and complete all of the other activities that were planned months ahead of time under the old survey process. Now your organization must be able to pull it together for a survey at a moment's notice, similar to the way it must snap into operation during a fire drill or a disaster.

In the first part of this chapter, we will approach the subject of preparation much like we would structure disaster response by simply defining who does what, who brings what, who calls whom, and who attends what. For it to come together, the unannounced survey plan must be practiced through several dry runs so that various people will have a chance to practice. After all, you don't know who will be available when the Joint Commission's extranet site is checked sometime before 7:30 a.m. and there it is: a posted notice that today is your survey.

Chapter 7

References for Planning

The most recent publication of the Joint Commission's *Survey Activity Guide* is available on the Joint Commission's Web site, and you should use it as your road map for developing your organization's unannounced survey plan. (In this chapter, I will reference the document but will not copy all of its information here, so be sure to refer to the document.)

In addition, the Accreditation Process chapter in the Joint Commission's standards manual outlines eligibility, the application, and many other topics that are necessary for survey preparation. Carefully review these references so that you understand the required components of a survey. Should you have any questions, contact the account executive The Joint Commission has assigned to your organization.

Sometime before your survey, the survey agenda specific for your organization will be posted on the Joint Commission's extranet site. Print the agenda for reference during the planning process. Unlike scheduled surveys, the agenda cannot be altered, but if adjustments need to be made on the morning of the survey, discuss them with the lead surveyor during the opening session.

Since 2007, the Joint Commission survey application as been in electronic format. If you have not previously been involved in completing your organization's application, go to the extranet and review its content. Familiarize yourself with the volume data and ensure that the information is accurate and current and that all services and facilities are included in the application. APR.01.02.01 requires the organization at any time, prior to or during a survey, to provide accurate information to avoid any challenge of falsification.

The accuracy of the application is also crucial to ensure that the correct mix of surveyor types and number of survey days is planned accordingly. Note that if your organization experiences changes in ownership, control, location, capacity, or services offered, you must notify The Joint Commission within 30 days after the change (per accreditation participation requirement APR.01.03.01). The statement regarding increases or decreases in volume in the "Handling Changes Affecting Information" section of the ACC chapter uses the term *significant change*. The definition of *significant* is not provided; to ensure that you are correct in your reporting, contact your account executive to determine whether volume changes are significant. Should the surveyors arrive and discover that information was left off the application, either intentionally or not, or that organizational updates were not provided, The Joint Commission may need to conduct another survey at a later date, which would delay your accreditation decision and possibly lead to additional survey charges.

> **Key Concept**
>
>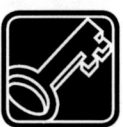
>
> A word of caution: If your organization intentionally omitted any information from the application and The Joint Commission is reasonably sure the organization submitted falsified or misrepresented information, The Joint Commission could recommend a preliminary denial of accreditation (accreditation decision rule PDA 03). This is serious, because if accreditation is denied, your organization is prohibited from participating in accreditation for one year. No deemed status would mean no billing of Medicare and Medicaid services.

Focus on the Front End, and Plan Carefully

In talking with many CEOs and other organizational leaders, you'll find that the one thing they all agree on is how vital the first half hour of the survey is to demonstrate to surveyors that you are prepared, organized, and ready. To assist you in making decisions regarding your survey preparation plan, a template is provided in Figure 7.1. As you are formulating your plan, you should assign at least one backup person to handle each task in the event of absences; some organizations may even choose to add a third person. This is only a template, and you should alter it to meet your organization's needs.

Chapter 7

Figure 7.1 ■ Checklist for Unannounced Joint Commission Survey Plan

Monitoring for Survey Notice: _____ **Backup:** _____

Check-off	Daily at 7:30 a.m., access the Joint Commission Connect Web site at *www.jointcommission.org*. Enter your password and hospital ID; select Notification of Scheduled Events.
	When notification of survey is posted:
❏	1. Alert switchboard to announce the survey and perform e-mail blast
❏	2. Alert _____ (sometimes house supervisor) to initiate page to executives and key personnel, including backups
	Print:
❏	1. Introductory letter authorizing the surveyors' presence for an unannounced survey
❏	2. Surveyor names, pictures, and biographies
❏	3. Agenda, if not already printed
❏	4. Priority focus processes (PFP), if not already printed
	Immediately distribute:
❏	1. Copy of surveyor names and pictures to front desk/switchboard staff
❏	2. Copy of agenda to administration to schedule meeting rooms
❏	3. All original printouts to designated survey coordinator

RESPONSES to page for setup

Check-off	Security officer and environmental services on duty:
❏	1. Unlock _____ room
❏	2. Tidy room, if necessary
❏	3. Notify _____ if alternative room should be considered (Internet access, phone, secured room, access to printer)
	Maintenance: _____ **Backup:** _____
❏	1. Check outlets, temperature, etc. in _____ room
❏	2. Notify _____ if alternative room should be considered
	Information services: _____ **Backup:** _____
❏	1. Ensure that Internet service is functional in _____ room
❏	2. Provide pass codes for surveyors to access the Internet
❏	3. Notify _____ if alternative room should be considered

Figure 7.1 ■ Checklist for Unannounced Joint Commission Survey Plan (Cont.)

RESPONSES to page for setup (Cont.)

Check-off	Backup:
☐	1. Retrieve *Unannounced Joint Commission Supplies* from location _____
☐	2. Take surveyor folders to _____ room
☐	3. Insert copy of agenda and PFP obtained from Joint Commission extranet into each surveyor folder if not already present

	_____ Backup: _____
☐	1. Obtain inpatient census and schedules for surgery, cardiac cath, and endoscopy
☐	2. Obtain visit schedule for home care, dialysis, etc.
☐	3. Deliver to _____ for surveyor review session
☐	4. Daily, obtain census and schedules and provide to each surveyor

	Director of food and nutritional services: _____ **Backup:** _____
☐	1. Prepare and deliver predetermined beverages, snacks, and menus to _____ room
☐	2. Prepare beverages for opening conference
☐	3. Ensure that food items are available for lunch choices listed on the surveyor menu

	Administration support staff: _____
☐	1. Cancel meetings that conflict with survey agenda
☐	2. Based on the agenda, reserve rooms for the survey, prioritizing day one:
☐	a. Opening conference
☐	b. Special issue resolution
☐	c. Daily briefing
☐	d. Infection control system tracer
☐	e. Data use system tracer
☐	f. Medication management system tracer
☐	g. Environment of care—review of management plans and group discussion
☐	h. Emergency management tracer
☐	i. Medical staff credentialing and privileging
☐	j. Competence assessment process
☐	k. Exit briefing with CEO
☐	l. Organization exit conference

Figure 7.1 ■ Checklist for Unannounced Joint Commission Survey Plan (Cont.)

RESPONSES to page for document delivery to the surveyor workroom if not already stored in centralized location:

❏ Performance improvement data from past 12 months: _____
   Backup: _____
   Location: _____

❏ Infection control data from past 12 months: _____
   Backup: _____
   Location: _____

❏ Core measures data: _____ Backup: _____
   Location: _____

❏ Medical record delinquency rates: _____ Backup: _____
   Location: _____

In response to page, retrieve documents for review by the life safety surveyor

❏ Environment of care: _____ Backup: _____
   Location: _____

❏   1. Environment of care meeting minutes (past 12 months)

❏   2. Environment of care data

❏   3. *Statement of Conditions*

❏   4. Plans for improvement (may be extranet accessible)

In response to page, set up the command center

❏ Primary: _____ Backup: _____
   Admin. asst.: _____ Backup: _____
   Add'l. staff: _____ Backup: _____
   Location: _____

❏   1. Ensure that two working phones are available

❏   2. Ensure that two computers with printer connection are available

❏   3. Reference manuals: standards manual, hardcopy policy book, telephone lists (two), etc.

❏   4. Escort supplies: clipboards, escort documentation worksheets, pens, sticky notes

❏   5. Message logs

Figure 7.1 ■ Checklist for Unannounced Joint Commission Survey Plan (Cont.)

ARRIVAL OF SURVEY TEAM at 8 a.m., Day 1:

Check-off	Front desk/switchboard staff: _____
☐	1. Verify identity of survey team by comparing Joint Commission picture ID to printed Joint Commission Connect information
☐	2. Telephone administrative office: [enter number here; if no answer, what is the next step?]
	Administrative assistant: _____
☐	1. Escort survey team to designated meeting room: _____ Backup room: _____
☐	2. Offer beverages
☐	3. Provide surveyors with location of restroom

SURVEYOR PLANNING SESSION, 8–9 a.m.

Review of documents; surveyors only

PREPARE FOR OPENING CONFERENCE (during surveyor planning session)

☐	1. Retrieve tent cards with attendee names from (*Unannounced Supplies*)			
☐	2. Distribute prepared organizational fact sheet to executive attendees			
☐	3. Confirm presence of surveyor escorts			
☐	Physician	1.	2.	3.
☐	Nurse	1.	2.	3.
☐	Administrator	1.	2.	3.
☐	Life safety	1.	2.	3.
☐	Other	1.	2.	3.

OPENING CONFERENCE/ORIENTATION TO ORGANIZATION, 9–10 a.m.

☐	1. Finalize agenda with surveyors
☐	2. Send agenda to department directors/supervisors: _____

> **Figure 7.1 ■ Checklist for Unannounced Joint Commission Survey Plan (Cont.)**
>
> For assistance in selecting participants, see suggestions in *Survey Activity Guide,* January 2009, Joint Commission Connect extranet.
>
> **WORKSHEET TO PREPLAN ATTENDEES AT SPECIFIC SURVEY SESSIONS**
>
> | Check-off | For life safety building tour |
> |---|---|
> | ❏ | Plant operations director |
> | ❏ | |
> | ❏ | |
> | ❏ | |
>
> | | **Environment of care session   Room: _____** |
> |---|---|
> | ❏ | Plant operations |
> | ❏ | Emergency management |
> | ❏ | Biomedical |
> | ❏ | Environmental safety |
> | ❏ | Security |
>
> | | **Emergency management session   Room: _____** |
> |---|---|
> | ❏ | |
> | ❏ | |
> | ❏ | |
> | ❏ | |
>
> | | **Medical staff credentialing and privileging   Room: _____** |
> |---|---|
> | ❏ | Medical staff coordinator |
> | ❏ | Credentials committee chair |
> | ❏ | Vice president of medical affairs |
> | ❏ | Medical staff president |
>
> | | **System tracer–data use   Room: _____** |
> |---|---|
> | | VP/director of performance improvement |
> | | Participants involved in most recent Failure Modes and Effects Analysis |
> | | Staffing effectiveness preparers |
> | | Participants in data provided for data review session |

Figure 7.1 ■ Checklist for Unannounced Joint Commission Survey Plan (Cont.)

WORKSHEET TO PREPLAN ATTENDEES AT SPECIFIC SURVEY SESSIONS

Check-off	System tracer—medication management Room: _____
☐	Pharmacy representatives
☐	Nursing representatives
☐	

System tracer—infection control   Room: _____

- ☐ Infection control practitioner
- ☐ Laboratory representative on infection control committee
- ☐

Competency assessment process   Room: _____

- ☐ VP human resources
- ☐ Educator
- ☐

Leadership session   Room: _____

☐ CEO ☐ EVP/COO ☐ CFO ☐ VP PI ☐ VP PCS ☐ VP APS ☐ VP HR
☐ CNO ☐ CIO ☐ Accreditation specialist ☐ ☐ ☐

Special issue resolution   Room: _____

- ☐
- ☐
- ☐

Daily briefing   Room: _____

- ☐
- ☐
- ☐

CEO exit briefing   Room: _____

- ☐ CEO

Organization exit conference   Room: _____

- ☐
- ☐
- ☐
- ☐

Because your time to enact your plan is extremely limited after you learn that this is day one of your survey, it is important that you check the extranet site promptly each workday at 7:30 a.m.

> **Success Story**
>
> 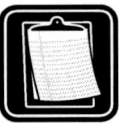 Some organizations have chosen to forego site checking until their 18-month survey window opens. This prevents staff members from becoming complacent with the task. Information from the field tells us that early surveys based on high Strategic Surveillance System scores have not occurred in 2009. For client hospitals surveyed in 2009, surveyors are arriving between 7:45 a.m. and 8:10 a.m.

Formulating a survey plan will require input from many areas. Because you know your hospital's culture and what works best, determine whether this should be a group task or whether it's best for the accreditation specialist to prepare a draft plan, with subsequent review by organizational leaders. Whichever approach you use, begin the following tasks:

1. Assign individuals who are already on-site by 7:15 a.m. and who can act under pressure to check the Web site.

2. Identify the methods of notifying leadership, key individuals, and the staff of the survey. Consider mass paging, mass e-mails, overhead announcements, and a telephone tree to reach everyone.

3. Determine who will print the items from the extranet. It may be the same person who initially checked the extranet, or because this person may be busy notifying others you may choose another person to perform the task. For backup, list an additional person who can be called to assist. Print the following items from the extranet:

    – Introductory letter legitimizing the survey
    – Surveyor names, pictures, and biographies
    – Agenda, if not already printed
    – Priority focus processes, if not already printed

4. Determine who will deliver the surveyor names and pictures to the entry point of your hospital for use in validating the surveyors' identities, deliver an agenda to the administrative assistant scheduling rooms, and take the original printed items to the survey coordinator.

> **Key Concept**
>
>
>
> If the surveyors walk up to the front desk before 8 a.m., will the desk be staffed? If not, where would the surveyors wander next? As previously stated, in 2009, surveyors generally arrived between 7:45 a.m. and 8:10 a.m.; however, most usually arrived before 8 a.m. to allow time to be escorted to their workroom and settle into their surroundings. Think this process through very carefully—you do not want surveyors to arrive to an unstaffed area and subsequently begin surveying as stated in the *Survey Activity Guide.*

5. Designate a surveyor workroom. Consider selecting a room that is adjacent to administration or the performance improvement department. This allows administrative assistants to be readily available to handle any special requests of the surveyors, and from a hospital perspective, surveyors can be kept in close view. The workroom should have a table and chairs with workspace adequate for the expected number of surveyors based on your organization's posted agenda, a telephone, and Internet connection capability. Doors to the room must lock, because surveyors have laptops, personal belongings, other valuable possessions, and confidential information to secure.

> **Field Experience**
>
>
>
> Do not put the surveyors in the room that you wish to use for the opening session/orientation. You want to be able to set up that room without having surveyors to work around. First impressions are lasting, so ensure that the people in position of initial contact are instructed to greet the surveyors, validate their identification, and offer them a place to sit while awaiting their designated escort.

6. Assign an individual to be accountable for assembling surveyor folders and keeping them concurrently updated. Often, the accreditation specialist assumes this responsibility. Because surveyors tend to make notes on some documents and often wish to reference them at another time during the survey, we have found that surveyors appreciate a preassembled folder that contains the following:

- Organizational chart with names of leadership
- Names of the organization's key contacts (three or four); this may be a main number to a command center, which we will discuss later
- List of hospital floors and types of services provided on each
- List of all sites, on and off campus, that are eligible for survey, and services provided at each site; include mileage from the hospital
- Agenda
- Primary focus areas (most recent)

> **Key Concept**
>
>
>
> Obtain and label a plastic storage tub as "Joint Commission Survey Supplies." Determine where this will be located for retrieval on survey day and store the surveyor folders and other items in this tub.

7. Determine who will retrieve the aforementioned supplies and deliver them to the surveyor workroom on the morning of the survey.

8. Prepare for the surveyors' orientation to the organization ahead of time and store all needed materials for this session with your unannounced-survey supplies. The opening session is to be interactive, and prepared PowerPoint presentations are not necessary; in fact, some surveyors discourage them. If you choose, prepare a brief presentation (no longer than 10 minutes) that provides an overview of the organization. Ask the lead surveyor what his or her preference is regarding a presentation versus a discussion. A presentation should include the types of information displayed in Figure 7.2 and be presented by the CEO or designee. The fact sheet is designed to be a cheat sheet for attendees to use when answering typical questions asked by surveyors. Prepare a fact sheet ahead of time and store it with the unannounced-survey supplies.

9. Utilize the planning worksheet and determine the appropriate attendees for the formalized group sessions and system tracers listed in Figure 7.3.

Figure 7.2 ■ Sample Fact Sheet

[Hospital name]

Demographics

- Ownership history
- Licensed beds
- Occupied beds
- Emergency department visits
- Number of deliveries
- Inpatient and outpatient services
- Clinical service groups with the highest volumes
- Pharmacy hours of operation
- Facilities included in the survey other than the hospital
- Number of medical staff members
- Type and number of allied health practitioners

Description of medical records

- Patient care areas using a paper record
- Where an electronic record is utilized
- Presence of computerized order entry

Other key information if asked by the surveyors (keep it brief on this fact sheet)

- Mission, vision, goals, and current strategic initiatives
- List of contractual clinical services
- List of types of students trained at your facility: medical students, residents, nursing, radiology, lab, etc.
- Organization's top primary focus areas
- Title of most recent FMEA; who will present if asked
- How the leaders prioritize quality and safety initiatives
- National patient safety goals; how adherence is measured

Chapter 7

Figure 7.3 ■ Survey Activities

- Opening conference/orientation to your organization
- Life safety building tour
- Environment of care session
- Emergency management session
- Medical staff credentialing and privileging
- System tracer—data use
- System tracer—medication management
- System tracer—infection control
- Competency assessment process
- Leadership session
- Daily briefing
- CEO briefing
- Organization exit conference

10. Identify the individuals who will serve as surveyor escorts. See Figure 7.4 for a listing of duties. As noted on the planning worksheet, select backups to cover for absences. An escort should be familiar both with the units the surveyor will most likely visit and the subject matter of his or her assignment and should also be able to locate units throughout the hospital. Prepare a list of phone and beeper numbers that each escort might need and store them with the unannounced-survey supplies for ready access prior to beginning tracers.

Field Experience

Limit the number of people accompanying the surveyors to just one escort. Plan to include the department manager upon arrival. A larger number of people is unyielding and inefficient and may irritate the surveyors.

Figure 7.4 ■ Surveyor Escort Duties

Duties:

- Accompany surveyor to selected area; never leave surveyor alone
- Record surveyors' questions and staff members' responses
- Document names of employees and physicians interviewed during tracers
- During tracers, record patient name and medical record; for efficiency, place a patient sticker on escort documentation worksheet
- Alert command center of focus/issues identified
- Report surveyor requests to command center
- Submit documentation worksheets at lunch and end of day to command center

11. Decide whether a centralized command center is to be used during the survey. A command center functions as a central clearinghouse for fielding inquiries and providing assistance with organizing escorts, retrieving documents requested by surveyors, and promoting readiness for system tracer sessions. Figure 7.5 shows an example of duties typical of a command center. Avoid using the accreditation specialist to lead the command center. This position tends to be pulled in multiple directions, and the command center staff needs to be focused on supporting escorts and surveyor requests. Consider adding to the command center staff an administrative assistant who has worked closely on survey readiness. Select another individual to work in the command center so that two people are in attendance at all times. Because one or the other may not be in town during the survey, have two other people trained to step in as backups.

12. If you choose to have a command center, decide where you will locate it. At least two telephones should be available to ensure that calls are answered at all times; an additional third line may be needed for larger facilities hosting more surveyors.

13. Determine the location for conducting a tracer in each patient care unit. This is particularly important when the medical record is electronic or when it is a hybrid of hard-copy and electronic documents. Don't expect the surveyors to sit at the nurses' station and ask candid questions about patient care. Select a room with adequate seating and a functioning computer. The use of the staff's break room should be discouraged, as it generally has that lived-in look and repetitive interruptions often occur. Don't overlook the possibility of using an empty patient room by pulling in chairs and a computer on wheels.

Figure 7.5 ■ Typical Command Center Duties

Survey Command Center

Telephone #1: _____

Telephone #2: _____

Location: _____

Duties:

- Each morning by 7:30 a.m., obtain and assemble copies of daily census and operating room (OR) schedules for each surveyor:
  - Census should include patient name, location, admitting diagnosis, and admission date or length of stay
  - OR schedules should have patient name, location, and procedure being performed
- Deliver copies to surveyor workroom by 7:45 a.m.
- Serve as the resource for surveyor requests for documents not readily available during tracer activities; review documents before submission to surveyors
- Receive, record, and communicate messages to surveyor escorts and other staff members as needed and as appropriate
- When possible, call ahead to departments as survey team moves through the facility (including ambulatory sites)
- Transcribe escort notes and track common issues on whiteboard each day
- Obtain staff and physician names identified during tracers and facilitate retrieval of employee human resources/department manager files and physician credential files by notifying appropriate individuals to review files (human resources and medical staff office)
- Prepare and send out communication to staff members as requested
- Verify attendee readiness for system tracers prior to start of sessions; arrange for replacements as needed
- Prepare list of needs, concerns, and activities for discussion at daily hospital survey team debriefing
- Obtain medical records as requested by survey team; preview if time allows

Define Expected Responses Following Survey Notification

1. **Security officer and environmental service worker:** It is always wise to have a representative from environmental services inspect the room designated for surveyors to ensure that the room is tidy. You don't want to discover at the last minute that the room you planned to use was not cleared of food and materials from the previous night's meeting. Security will have the keys and be available to open rooms that may be locked and inaccessible.

2. **Maintenance:** Ensure that the temperature is acceptable and that lighting and outlets are functional; generally inspect the room.

3. **Information services:** Access to the Internet is not listed as a requirement; however, surveyors often request it. A designee should have determined the availability of wireless or cable connections at the time the room was selected. A designated representative from information services should proceed to the surveyor workroom and confirm that Internet access is operational, and if necessary, give the surveyors the access code.

4. **Food services:** Preplan the amount and type of beverages to be needed in the surveyor workroom and the opening conference. Light snacks should be provided for the surveyors. Following notification, the items should be delivered to the surveyor workroom and subsequently to the room chosen for the opening conference at 9 a.m.

> **Field Experience**
>
>
>
> One thing that surveyors seem to like is being offered a menu of lunch options early each morning. Allow the surveyors to select from three or four options of stock food items that they prefer or that are compatible with their food allergies, special diets, and so on. The menu should be developed ahead of time and delivered each morning with the beverages.

5. **Administrative support staff:** Consider choosing at least two people for the tasks in this section, because they can be occurring simultaneously:
   - Contact designated escorts to ensure that they are on campus. Based on the agenda, begin reserving rooms for the meetings for the first survey day. Cancel meetings that

may conflict with the survey agenda and the persons who need to attend. Reserve meeting rooms for the remainder of the survey days.

– Set up the room chosen for the opening conference/orientation. With the surveyors initially reviewing documents for an hour, this allows time to summon the appropriate people for the opening conference and to set up the room. Copy the agenda for the opening conference attendees and distribute it throughout the organization via an e-mail batch or fax.

Key Concepts

Use placards for the opening conference to help the surveyors match the names of leaders with their faces. Also include each person's functional area of responsibility on the placard. Store these with the other unannounced-survey supplies. Store some blank placards for use in case additional surveyors or other attendees are present. You can also prepare placards for the other sessions.

6. **Command center staff:** Obtain copies of the inpatient census and schedules for surgery, cardiac cath, and endoscopy to be delivered to the surveyor workroom.

Field Experience

The census should include each patient's diagnosis and admission date. As a consultant conducting mock surveys, I have been provided with documents that staff members were unable to decipher, so make sure your documents are clear. Also, when asked about units or floors, do not respond with "3 West" or "the Blue Unit." Specify the type of patient cared for in the unit, such as medical or orthopedics. If you need to write this information by hand onto each floor census, do so to facilitate surveyor comprehension.

A major function of the command center is to field telephone calls. To aid staff members in tracking calls, Figure 7.6 provides a sample phone log.

Figure 7.6 ■ Sample Phone Log

The Joint Commission Command Center Messages

Date: _____

Message For	Message From	Time	Initials/Comments

Chapter 7

During your next survey, be prepared for a request for closed or open records. As published in the October 2009 issue of *Perspectives,* for organizations seeking Joint Commission accreditation for deemed status purposes, surveyors are required to look at a specific number of medical records based on the organization's average daily census (ADC). Ten percent of the ADC, minimally 30 inpatient records, must be reviewed. Many of these will be done in tracers, but the volume will depend on the number of surveyors. Small general hospitals, not specifically defined, are subjected to 20 medical record reviews.

7. **Departments throughout the organization:** When the survey is announced, take a tour through your department and look at it through the eyes of a surveyor. Remove clutter from desktops, store equipment out of the hallways, and ensure that medical gas shut-off valves and fire pulls are not obstructed, doors are not propped open, and medication rooms are locked. Remind staff members to carry on with patient care as usual. Ensure that all employees present are wearing their name badges.

Practice Your Plan

Conduct unannounced survey drills

After you've formulated your plan for responding to an unannounced survey, it's time to practice and train the participants, similar to the process used for fire drills. Practice activating your plan by having the "surveyors" arrive at your facility. It is imperative that this goes smoothly to avoid rattling the confidence of the participants and to avoid setting the stage negatively for the remainder of the survey. First impressions are lasting, so make sure the initial contact people who will potentially serve as greeters are instructed in their roles to greet the surveyors, validate their identification, and offer them a place to sit while awaiting their designated escort. Figure 7.7 describes greeters' duties. Enlist the help of several hospital volunteers to serve as surveyors by arriving to the front desk and stating, "Hello, we are here to assist you in preparing for your Joint Commission survey. Please proceed as if we were the actual surveyor." Obtain the volunteers' feedback and their perception of staff member awareness in terms of what to implement, customer service, and promptness of implementation. Assess how rapidly the call was initiated from the arrival location to the key contact person(s) on your plan. Determine whether all the required documents and surveyor folders were delivered to the designated surveyor workroom. The items listed in this chapter as responses to notification of a survey should be assessed for completion of tasks and for timeliness.

Figure 7.7 ■ Greeters' Duties

Joint Commission Greeters

Greeters are the first person(s) to greet the surveyors when they arrive on the first day of the survey. This is usually around 7:45 a.m. The surveyors could enter at either of these entrances:

_____
(fill in entrance here)

_____
(fill in entrance here)

Potential Greeters

Administrative supervisors, security guards, parking attendants, switchboard operators, volunteers

Duties of Greeters

- Monitor entrances on morning of survey announcement
- Greet surveyors upon arrival
- Ask surveyors for identification and verify with extranet printout
- Offer seating while awaiting escort
- Contact _____ to escort surveyors to _____ workroom

Key Concepts

If you conduct this practice as a paper drill only, you will not achieve the timeliness needed on the morning of the survey. Hold a drill when key personnel are not available and backup staff members need to step in and take charge. For example, could your organization pull it together if you, the survey coordinator, were on vacation 2,000 miles away? They should be able to.

Practice the interview sessions and system tracers

Schedule a practice session for the sessions listed in Figure 7.3. Some may think this is unnecessary and a bit overkill, but practicing will help put the participants at ease. Plus, it provides you, the accreditation specialist, with an opportunity to coach them on the best responses.

Provide each participant with a description of his or her assigned session as found in the *Survey Activity Guide*. Walk the participants through the topics to be discussed and have them practice their responses. Encourage more than one participant to answer each question, because you can't be sure who will be present on the day of the actual survey. Promote discussion and suggestions for additional answers or examples of standards compliance. Watch for periods of uncertainty, as you may learn as much from the group's silence as you do from long-winded responses.

> **Key Concept**
>
>
>
> The leadership session is held toward the end of the survey for a reason. Listen very carefully at the daily briefings and the subjects presented at the special issue resolution. The subjects of these sessions often end up being the basis of the questions presented to leadership to learn how the subject was identified, what actions leaders implemented, and so forth.

Don't waste time requiring staff members to memorize answers to questions that surveyors might ask. It's more important for them to be comfortable with the tracer process and have appropriate etiquette with the surveyors. Advise staff members to admit nervousness. The surveyors understand that this may be their first survey. Also, tell staff members to ask surveyors to restate any questions that they feel are unclear.

Conduct an orientation for the surveyor escorts

Tell all staff members the phone number and location of the surveyor workroom, and record the number on the bottom of the escort documentation worksheets, as shown in Figure 7.8.

Figure 7.8 ■ Escort Documentation Worksheet

Date: _____ Escort name: _____

Surveyor name: _____

Command center phone #s: _____

Location	Staff/Physician/Patient Interviewed/ Record Reviewed	Questions Surveyors Ask/Issues Identified/Pertinent Observations

Please return completed worksheets at lunchtime and at the end of the day to the command center.

Review the escort duties shown in Figure 7.4. Instruct the surveyor escorts to record the name and number of each medical record reviewed. A simple way to accomplish this is to obtain a patient label from the record.

Record surveyor comments and take sufficient notes to summarize discussions with leadership and the accreditation coordinator at the close of survey activities and the surveyors' exit each day. By reviewing the surveyors' verbalized findings, leadership can initiate further discussions or clarifications with the surveyors during the next morning's briefing or during the special issues resolution session later in the day.

Distribute information regarding the command center

Instruct department managers and staff members to contact the command center with requests for documents, special requests of the surveyors, and names of any employees identified for competency review or practitioners identified for credentialing review.

List the types of problems and issues that need to be brought to your immediate attention, such as a major deviation from the readiness plan, changes in the agenda, disruptive behavior (surveyor or staff member), and surveyor statements of "conditional or predenial of accreditation."

Day of Survey

The Joint Commission extranet site says today is the day. Stick to your predefined rollout plan. Trying to be creative at the last minute, while you're under time constraints and survey stress, is an invitation for failure.

Following the surveyors' arrival, the preliminary planning session will begin

This 8 a.m. session is often referred to as "document review," but the actual name is "preliminary planning session." Remember, during this session the surveyors begin to review documents to become acquainted with your organization. Surveyors do not arrive with an organizational resume and multitudes of organizational data. They rely on the information provided by the facility.

So to set the stage and to demonstrate that the organization is ready for the survey, individuals designated to deliver documents to the surveyor workroom should do so promptly. Do not dawdle; the surveyors are skilled and will move quickly through their initial folder of information. If the required documents are not available in a timely manner, the surveyors may proceed to patient care areas and begin individual tracer activities.

Additional documents that you should have readily available because surveyors often request them are discussed in Chapter 8 under the heading "Individual Tracer Activities." Do not offer or provide these additional documents to the surveyors until they request them.

> **Field Experience**
>
>
> If surveyors arrive with a list of documents that are not included in the *Survey Activity Guide,* do not let that throw you off your stride. Simply explain that you will acquire the documents as soon as possible. Then contact the command center for their assistance. Ease the focus back to the required documents that are currently available for their review.

After the opening conference/orientation, the surveyors will be ready to select individual patients for tracer activities. The surveyors may ask for assistance. This is an excellent opportunity to introduce their escorts and have the escorts assist in tracer selection.

As the surveyors begin their tracer activities, do not try to guess where they may travel and attempt to notify staff members in advance. Not only is this a waste of time, but covert ploys such as this should no longer be necessary now that your organization is practicing continuous survey readiness.

> **Key Concept**
>
>
> As issues are identified, do *not* scramble in an attempt to fix things during the survey. At the time of the survey, "it is what it is." Also, by attempting to fix something, the organization has inadvertently accepted that something was wrong. This hampers the clarification process following the survey. All surveyors participate in preparing the survey report. Once the report is completed, an exit briefing is held for approximately 15 minutes with the most senior leader present in the organization.

Chapter 7

Exit Briefing

During the exit briefing, the following occurs:

- A report of requirements for improvement (RFI) is presented

- Any concerns about the report are discussed

- The senior leader decides whether an organizational exit conference will occur, and if so, whether copies of the report are to be distributed

Organizational exit conference

The senior leader determines who will attend the organizational exit conference, but generally it includes the individuals who attended the opening conference plus organizationwide managerial staff members. This varies greatly based on the survey outcome, logistics, and size of the organization.

If desired, the organization also is responsible for preparing photocopies of the report for distribution.

During this 30-minute session, the surveyors provide the following:

- Standard compliance issues and RFIs

- If applicable, the process for submitting evidence of standards compliance and measures of success

- "What Happens After Your Survey" brochure

Once the survey activities have concluded, the surveyors will begin to aggregate their findings. Absent from the report will be the potential accreditation decision. Their report is preliminary and the final report will be posted to the extranet within 10 business days.

Attendees, as determined by the organization, are informed of the standard compliance issues and the RFIs. This session concludes after approximately 30 minutes.

TEST YOUR KNOWLEDGE

1. You have been asked to assist in assigning staff members to participate in the data use system tracer. Select the best choices for this task from the following positions:

    A. Chief nursing officer
    B. Performance improvement director
    C. Core measures abstractor
    D. Pharmacist who evaluates medication management

    1. A, B, C
    2. B, C, D
    3. A, C, D
    4. All of the above

Answer: 2. Even though the chief nursing officer may be familiar with many data collection projects, his or her time is usually focused on tracer activities and he or she is not in attendance at the data use session.

2. True or false: Surveyors are not allowed to arrive at the organization for a survey prior to 8 a.m.

Answer: False. Surveyors may arrive anytime after the notice of survey is posted on the extranet, and the notice must be posted by 7:30 a.m. local time. In actuality, most surveyors arrive just before 8 a.m.

3. Match the most appropriate session for the listed personnel to attend during an on-site survey.

    A. Risk manager
    B. Nursing educator
    C. Emergency department director
    D. COO

    1. Daily briefing
    2. Emergency management session
    3. Data use session
    4. Competence assessment process

Answer: A. 3
          B. 4
          C. 2
          D. 1

CHAPTER 8

The Challenges of Required Written Documentation

When the *Comprehensive Accreditation Manual for Hospitals* (*CAMH*) refreshed core was published in January 2009, a positive surprise was the inclusion of a tab near the back of the book labeled "RWD." Within the tab is a listing of all elements of performance (EP) with a circle D icon that require written documentation, sorted by chapter and standard number. The introduction of the chapter describes the "D" icon as identifying, in either paper or electronic format, documentation such as:

- A policy or procedure
- Bylaws
- Quality control testing data
- Medication labels
- A written plan
- A license
- Performance improvement reports
- Meeting minutes
- Material safety data sheets

One of the drawbacks of the RWD chapter is the lack of a narrative explanation of each EP. It would take hours to look at each of these items, and without the knowledge of the EP content, this chapter isn't very helpful. To be able to use this as a checklist and as a tool to perform an inventory of documents, we can thank **Jodi Eisenberg, MHA, CPHQ, CPMSM, CSHA,** manager of clinical accreditation and policy management at Northwestern Memorial Hospital in Chicago. Jodi took the time to prepare a spreadsheet for each chapter. She was willing to share this for your use, and a full copy of the checklist is included in the appendix. Within the spreadsheet, each chapter appears on a separate sheet and is labeled on the tabs at the bottom of the screen.

To provide you with a sneak preview, Figure 8.1 displays the category D EPs with the appropriate chapter of the *CAMH*. Note that the sheet groups data by document type, with policies at the top and plans at the bottom. A column is provided to enter the name of the document or type of documentation and when the item was last updated.

Figure 8.1 ■ Information Management Circle D Elements of Performance

Chapter	Standard	Element of Performance	Content	Hospital Policy	Responsible Party	Last Update
IM	02.01.01	1	Written policy addressing the privacy of health information			
IM	02.01.03	1	Written policy addressing the security of health information, including access, use, and disclosure			
IM	02.01.03	2	Written policy addressing the integrity of health information against loss, damage, unauthorized alteration, unintentional change, and accidental destruction			
IM	02.01.03	3	Written policy addressing the intentional destruction of health information			
IM	02.02.03	1	Written policies addressing data capture, display, transmission, and retention			
Chapter	**Standard**	**Element of Performance**	**Content**	**Plan**	**Responsible Party**	**Last Update**
IM	01.01.03	1	Written plan for managing interruptions to its information processes (paper-based, electronic, or a mix of paper-based and electronic)			

> **Key Concept**
>
>
> You can print these sheets and provide them to chapters or focus teams during the internal assessment, so they can use them to document the evidence they used to score a circle D EP. At that time, the location of documents, which is often a challenge in itself, could be determined, and if desired, an additional column could be added to the spreadsheet.

If you're working through the required category D items and you find that an item is not represented in a policy or guideline, resist the urge to draft another document. Research an existing document that addresses the same topic and add to it. In fact, one of the side benefits of cross-referencing documents to the Joint Commission requirements is an opportunity to merge policies and procedures, especially department-specific ones that restate the organization's administrative policy.

> **Field Experience**
>
>
> A common question from clients concerns The Joint Commission's requirement for frequency of policy review. Many years ago, it was recommended that policies be reviewed at least every three years, but that is long gone. At the time of this writing, there are no references to policy review, but state health departments may have regulations that address policies. Should a surveyor raise the issue of whether a policy is current, your oranization's policy regarding policies may be requested.

Even though we know that the days of only document review are long gone, we also know that tracer activities often generate inquires regarding expected procedures and the surveyor will ask for supporting documents. Don't underestimate the importance of documents as they are still key evidence to demonstrate integration of requirements into operations and functions.

We also know that many of the functional programs, such as infection control, emergency management, and performance improvement, are operationalized via a written plan describing the purpose, scope, and processes. So it seems an organization should minimally have the circle D documents referenced in the EPs. Prepare with the end in mind. If your organization has conducted a thorough and

Chapter 8

credible internal assessment of standards compliance as we discussed in Chapter 5, many of the category D documents should have been reviewed. One of an accreditation specialist's top priorities should be to *influence* the hospital's development and maintenance of documents that are simply stated, well organized, and readily retrievable for unannounced accreditation surveys.

As we discussed in Chapter 7, specific documents should be readily available for the surveyor preliminary planning session, also dubbed "document review," that will occur shortly after the surveyors arrive at your hospital. The required documents are identified in the Joint Commission's *Survey Activity Guide,* which was most recently updated in January 2009 and is located on both the Joint Commission's Web site and its extranet.

At any time during survey activities, a surveyor may request to see a specific item, such as a policy, procedure, plan, or meeting minutes. These requests should be forwarded to the command center, where staff members will promptly retrieve the document and deliver it to the surveyor.

Field Experience

It is unrealistic to attempt to maintain current copies of required documents within a single binder for continuous survey readiness—you and your staff would be forever pushing papers and playing a game of seek-and-replace. Some organizations continue to attempt to assemble a notebook for each chapter of the standards manual, but this is an old survey preparedness modality that has proven to be burdensome and ineffective. Considering what has happened with the Standards Improvement Initiative, such notebooks would now have to be reorganized, and for what purpose?

The Required Documents: One by One

Organizational chart

Provide a simplistic display of leadership with the reporting departments or functions listed. It is very helpful to the surveyors if the name of the individual holding the position can be included.

> **Field Experience**
>
>
>
> Avoid multipage monstrosities that require analysis to determine where the CEO is listed. Surveyors are interested in the main organization, and if they have questions regarding detail, they will ask.

Name and number of the contact person who will assist the surveyors during survey

This person is generally the accreditation specialist. Depending on whether you have chosen to operate a command center, provide the phone number of an individual or the command center. Ensure that the number provided is always answered and does not ring to voicemail.

> **Key Concept**
>
>
>
> Post the name of the individual plus the phone number in the surveyor workroom. Have an adequate number of contact sheets available for all surveyors to carry with them. Do not provide the surveyors with a copy of your hospital's internal phone listing. This is an open invitation for a surveyor to contact department managers without the benefit of an escort available to monitor the inquiry and assist with the response.

Map of your organization

This item is listed as a requirement but is rarely used by surveyors. Life safety surveyors are interested in detailed blueprints and not simplistic maps. Blueprints may remain within the facilities department for use in that location. Feedback from recently surveyed hospitals indicated that surveyors found it was more helpful to receive a listing of the floors in the hospital and a description of which services were located on each floor.

List of all sites eligible for survey

When preparing this list, ensure that it exactly matches the e-App stored on the extranet. Contact your account executive for assistance. Keep this document simple. Because the surveyors will be traveling to selected locations, include the mileage from the hospital to each site. Off-site building names sometimes do not reveal the services provided there, so read on to identify a mechanism to aid the surveyors in learning the location of off-site services.

List of services provided at each site

> **Success Stories**
>
>
>
> One of the most useful examples of a document displayed by a client was a simple table listing the buildings in the left column and the services provided at each site in the right column. This is easy to read and useful to all surveyors.
>
> Avoid the use of acronyms that are known by staff members but will be confusing to surveyors. Referencing a floor as 3 South does not convey the types of patients cared for on that unit. Additional information such as business occupancy may be helpful if the document remains easy to read. Depict what buildings are on the main campus and which are located elsewhere.

Performance improvement data

Please note that this says *data*—not performance improvement *committee minutes*. Not only are large volumes of performance improvement committee meeting minutes for the past three years unnecessary, but you are also providing documents that will increase your exposure to information that could result in findings.

This is your opportunity to put forward the best examples of performance improvement data that your organization has generated. The decisions are yours on what you will select. Think about improvement projects that you are really proud of; something that made a difference in patient care.

> **Key Concept**
>
> Consider including some of the most commonly expected topics—for example, those listed in PI.01.01.01, such as medication errors, organ procurement rates, patient/employee satisfaction surveys, restraint usage, staffing effectiveness, patient flow, and core measures. In addition, the National Patient Safety Goals (NPSG) that require data collection—hand hygiene compliance, critical results reporting, and anticoagulation program evaluation—should also be included.

Whichever data are selected, it is imperative that they "tell the story" of quantifiable measures, data analysis, selection of correlated interventions for improvement, and subsequent remeasurement.

> **Field Experience**
>
> The most frequent shortcoming of performance improvement data is the lack of meaningful analysis. If the analysis is simply a restatement of the measurements, do not include it in your showcase materials unless the analysis can be enhanced. Analysis need not be scientific. Think of it as variation analysis: For process indicators, focus on noncompliance to the process. Divide the noncompliance into reasons why the process was not followed. Display the reasons in a pie chart or go back to Chapter 6 and check out the Pareto chart, which is perfect for variation analysis.

Infection-related data

Again, this says *data* and not *meeting minutes, annual narrative reports, infection control plans,* and so on. The same rules apply as with the performance improvement data, with the exception that the data displayed should be based on the prioritized risks identified in the annual risk assessment or based on the surveillance plan. All the other types of infection control documents will be subject to review during the infection control system tracer. Do not provide materials that are not requested.

Plenty of data should be generated with the newly implemented NPSGs for multidrug-resistant organisms, central line infection prevention, and surgical site infections. Compliance with the evidence-based guidelines and outcome measurements of infection rates could be included if the rules of analysis and correlated actions exist.

Environment of care data, Statement of Conditions (SOC), *and plans for improvement*

These documents are going to be reviewed by the life safety surveyor, who may or may not remain in the preliminary planning session. Many times, the life safety surveyor prefers to begin the building tour and review documents at a later point in time. Regardless, these items should be available, even if they are reviewed at a later time.

Regarding data, consider using the data that are typically presented during the environment of care committee meeting, such as injuries, security incidences, critiques of drills, and so forth.

Even though the *SOC* and plans for improvement are on the extranet, a printed copy should be available for review. It is not unheard of to have the information systems go down during a survey or the extranet be unavailable.

> **Field Experience**
>
>  When delivering these documents to the designated surveyor workroom, use a crate or cart. That way, if the life safety surveyor chooses to review the materials in the facilities department, he or she can easily take them there. This also removes these documents from the scrutiny of other surveyors, so do not leave them behind for later retrieval.

Environment of care meeting minutes

Surveyors will request 12 months' worth of environment of care meeting minutes, so do not provide three years' worth. Also, ensure that the most recent meeting materials are displayed behind the tab even if the minutes are not yet prepared. One of the most flagrant offenses is to provide 12 months' worth of minutes, with the most recent being more than six months old when the committee meets monthly.

>
> **Key Concept**
>
> Ensure that these minutes are concurrently organized and divided by tabs based on either the meeting dates or the month of the meetings. Failure to locate documents can be a real detriment during the environment of care evaluation, and surveyors are not always willing to wait for requested items to be located.

Patient lists

This topic includes the current census for all patient care units and scheduled procedures for the operating room, endoscopy suites, cardiac catheterization, and so forth. Take the time to assess how well these documents present to the reader. An inpatient census should include the patient care unit, patient's name, admission date, admitting diagnosis, and preferably the length of stay, even though it can be calculated from the admission date.

Various census types are often available from the mainframe software, so if your census does not include these elements, work with either information systems or the health information department to discuss alternative formats.

Do not forget to gather appointments and visit lists for off-site facilities. Surveyors may want to plan their day, and if home care is involved, home visits can be time-consuming.

>
> **Key Concept**
>
> If your census uses nomenclature of the patient care unit that only employees can decipher, such as "3W," prepare stickers that describe the type of unit and place these in the unannounced survey supply tub. On survey days, adhere these stickers to the census for an explanation of floor types, such as medical or OB/GYN.

Procedure schedules should include the name of the patient, procedure to be performed, time of the procedure, and second identifier used for patient identification. The same rules apply as before. Some surveyors like to plan their day so that they are available to watch at least the beginning of procedures to assess compliance to the Universal Protocol™. Therefore, you should watch procedures to observe how laterality is depicted. If your policy requires "right" or "left" to be spelled out, ensure that "rt." "lt." is not on the schedule.

>
> **Key Concept**
>
> The Universal Protocol begins at the time the decision is made to perform a procedure, and the next step is the schedule. Some surveyors scrutinize the schedule very carefully to determine how it supports the identification of the patient, the procedure to be performed, and whether laterality is involved.

>
> **Field Experience**
>
> Some clients have actually presented handwritten schedules during on-site assessments when their scheduling systems are electronic. When questioned about this, staff members stated that they did not know how to print the schedule, so as a substitute, they wrote out the schedule by hand each day. Prior to survey, look at your schedules through "another set of eyes" and make adjustments as needed to put your best foot forward.

Measures of success

Historically, this was the only component of your periodic performance review (PPR) that surveyors were allowed to view, and rarely did they remember to do so. With the changes in the PPR process under evaluation, it is possible that this material will no longer be on the required list.

The intent of the review was to validate that the methodology of data collection was properly performed and that the results were equal to what was reported. Perhaps this will be a portion of the "touch points" that we discussed in Chapter 4.

Documents typically requested for survey activities

It is recommended that documents that are often requested during other survey activities be readily available and be organized as part of routine operations. Once the survey is announced, you will have some time to inspect the documents and ensure that they are in proper order, but you will not have adequate time to search for missing documents or those that are not yet filed, which sometimes is an issue in the human resources department or the medical staff office.

Orientation to your organization

This is generally an interactive discussion between the surveyors and the leaders of the organization. However, surveyors often ask questions about numbers of physicians and allied health professionals, which clinical services are contracted, priority focus areas, clinical service groups, and what types of medical records will be encountered on the various units.

Because surveys are unannounced, employees who readily know the answers to these questions cannot be guaranteed to be present on survey day. For this reason, you should consider compiling a fact sheet. It can be prepared in advance, stored with your unannounced-survey supplies, and used as a reference by hospital leadership. (We have included a sample fact sheet in Figure 7.2.) Other requests for documents should be forwarded to the command center for retrieval.

Individual tracer activity

During tracers, staff members may be asked about their hospital's policy regarding turnaround times for referrals following an initial nursing assessment, pain assessment or reassessment, or another common request relating to restraints and expectations for monitoring restrained patients. If staff members are able to clearly articulate these requirements, the surveyor may forego a request for the written policy. If staff members stumble on their answers or provide answers that conflict with what the surveyor was told in another patient care unit, the policy will be requested.

Frequently requested policies should be readily available and current. It is recommended that the following policies be reviewed for adherence to the standards:

- Pain assessment
- Sedation/anesthesia preassessment
- Use of restraints and seclusion
- Informed consent
- Advance directives
- Tissue management
- Assessment and reassessment
- Medication orders
- Medication storage

- Fall prevention
- History and physical requirements

Competence assessment

At the time of competency review, surveyors will expect that the appropriate documents are contained within the human resources file or a departmental manager's file and that they are orderly. The following documents should be available for the personnel selected for review during this session:

- Job description.

- Primary source verification of licensure, certification, or registration if required by law to perform job duties.

- Verification of requirements listed in the Qualifications section of the job description, such as education, training, and so on, by a method defined by the hospital.

- Evidence of general orientation if hired within the past three years.

- Departmental orientation if hired within the past three years or if changed position within the hospital.

- Completion of competency prior to performing job duties if hired within the past three years or if changed position.

- Ongoing competency as defined by the hospital/department.

- Performance evaluations for the frequency defined by the organization for the past three years. The Joint Commission does not require documents to be located within any particular department. It is up to the hospital to decide where the documents will be filed. The important factor is to collect all of the information and have it ready promptly after the names of the personnel are provided.

Field Experience

Should you find that license verification or some other date-sensitive document is missing, do not try to correct the situation. This practice could be considered falsification of presented materials, as the document was not present in the file at the time the individual was selected for review. At survey time, it is what it is.

- A deal breaker for competency review is the inability to locate items in personnel files. It is imperative that personnel files be organized and that the staff members assigned to facilitate the session are knowledgeable of the hiring process and general orientation. Each surveyor has his or her own style of conducting competency review, but when staff members stumble with initial questions, the process becomes very stressful.

Medical Staff Credentialing and Privileging

Medical staff offices are usually meticulous in their file maintenance practices. Several vendors offer preprinted tabs and specially designed file folders to decrease the labor intensity of filing multiple documents. The time allotted for pulling credentialing files will not be generous enough to allow staff members to file loose items and organize a file that is in disarray. Therefore, each time a credentialing file is handled it should be examined for loose filing and items that are out of order.

Physicians and allied health practitioners, if processed through the medical staff office, will be selected for review during tracer activities. The following documents should be ready for review for each practitioner selected:

- Primary source verification of licensure
- Approved privileges or scope of practice for allied health practitioners
- Evidence of focused professional performance evaluation for practitioners appointed subsequent to January 1, 2008
- Ongoing professional performance evaluations
- Quality data for practitioners reappointed prior to January 1, 2008
- Primary source verification of education and training for appointments within the previous three years
- Peer recommendations

The same caution applies here as with personnel files: Do not attempt to supplement or perform verifications not previously included in the file. If the verification is complete but not yet filed, by all means retrieve the document if time allows.

> **Key Concept**
>
> The focused practitioner performance evaluation and the ongoing practitioner performance evaluation are under a microscope and will be evaluated by the physician surveyor. The document that describes these processes should be pulled and readily available should it be requested.

Program-specific tracer: Suicide prevention

During this tracer, occasionally surveyors will ask to see the materials offered to the patient for crisis management at the time of discharge. If this occurs, contact the individuals most often involved in this process for their assistance.

If staff members are unable to answer the surveyors' questions regarding screening for suicide risk, the request for the policy could occur.

Program-specific tracer: Patient flow

This tracer often includes a request to see past data collection, analysis, and actions taken to reduce the impact of patient flow problems. Corrective actions must be organizationwide and not focused only on the emergency department.

Environment of care session

As noted in the required documentation, the past 12 months' worth of the environment of care committee minutes are needed for this session. Additionally, the plans for safety, security, hazardous materials management, fire safety, medical equipment, and utilities will be reviewed. An annual review of the goals established for each plan and evidence of presentation to the board should be flagged for this session.

The hazards vulnerability analysis is a document that is often requested early in the review, and the surveyor uses the document to generate questions based on the most likely hazard to strike the hospital. This will also be a discussion point during the emergency management tracer.

The Environment of Care chapter requires a large amount of documentation of monitoring of equipment and functional areas; any of these types of documentation are subject to review.

If construction is occurring, be prepared to provide the infection control risk analysis to the environment of care surveyor. This risk assessment should not be confused with the annual risk assessment focusing on community risks and healthcare-associated infections (HAI) that is reviewed during the infection control system tracer.

By far, this review session includes more document and data review than any of the other survey activities. Adequate support staff members are needed to concurrently maintain documents; last-minute assembly is not possible for the environment of care session.

Emergency management tracer

The emergency management plans and hazardous vulnerability analysis will be a major part of this review. Variation exists among surveyors, but of late, scenarios of an emergency are described and staff members are asked to explain their roles and responsibilities.

Evidence of past drills and critiques will be requested with an emphasis on interventions for improvement.

Life safety building assessment

The *SOC* and the plans for improvement will be reviewed during this part of the survey. The building maintenance program, if established, will be requested. Blueprints of the buildings will be used to study layout and to assess arrangement of smoke compartments, location of any suites, and so on. If construction is occurring, the documentation of interim life safety measures will be reviewed and evaluated for compliance.

Data management system tracer

The data provided for surveyor review during the initial surveyor planning session will now be open for discussion. Attendees should be prepared to answer questions regarding the previously supplied data. A folder of the Failure Modes and Effects Analysis (FMEA), which is now required to be performed once every 18 months, should be available with an emphasis on how the improvements in process were measured following the FMEA. Data supporting after-implementation monitoring are a plus.

IC system tracer

One of the first documents usually requested is the annual risk assessment. Based on this assessment, evidence of prioritization of risks must be documented with formulated strategies to reduce the risk for each priority. Surveillance data aggregated into a report of HAIs should be ready for the surveyor's review. In addition, the following items are likely to be requested:

- Data regarding staff exposures to infectious disease

- Flu vaccination rates and planned interventions to increase these rates

- Beginning January 2010, data generated from the implementation of the following three NPSGs: central line–associated blood stream infections, multidrug-resistant organisms, and surgical site infections

- Actions taken as a result of surveillance and outcomes data

> **Key Concept**
>
>
>
> Typically, this tracer will continue in a patient care unit. The surveyor will be assessing the implementation of infection control practices showcased during the interview session.

TEST YOUR KNOWLEDGE

1. Which types of documents may be applicable to meeting circle D EPs?

   A. Performance improvement data
   B. Conflict of interest policy
   C. Infection control plan
   D. Ongoing profession practice evaluation data

   1. A, B, and D
   2. B, C, and D
   3. A, B, and C
   4. All of the above

Answer: 3. Data are a component of the ongoing profession practice evaluation data process, but it is the elements of performance labeled with the icon circle D that are listed in A, B and C.

2. True or false: Electronic records are a hindrance to the patient tracer process. It is suggested that documentation requested by the surveyor be promptly printed.

Answer: False. In fact, this is very false. More healthcare organizations are using electronic records than ever before. The key to a successful electronic tracer is to ensure that staff members are able to locate the appropriate screens that display the requested information.

3. During the data use session, which of the following would be the most appropriate to have prepared to display should the surveyor ask for examples of data improvement?

   A. The medication administration FMEA conducted three years ago
   B. Central line insertion checklist usage showing improvements from 50% to 75%
   C. A near miss with a credible root-cause analysis pending outcome data
   D. None of the above

   1. A and B
   2. A, B, and C
   3. C
   4. D

Answer: 4. The FMEA is too old and this might trigger questions regarding why a more recently FMEA is not being presented. Although progress is being made, the use of a checklist is a category C EP requiring 90% compliance. A root-cause analysis is incomplete without data to evaluate effectiveness. Go back to the drawing board and find other examples of data use that "tell the story."

CHAPTER 9

After-Survey Activities

Organizations surveyed in 2009 should have seen a timelier posting of their survey report to the Joint Commission extranet. Just as other changes came forth as a result of the Joint Commission reapplying for deemed status from the Centers for Medicare & Medicaid Services (CMS), the requirement for a 10-day turnaround time was levied. This seems only fair; after all, organizations seeking accreditation have strict time frames to abide by, so why shouldn't The Joint Commission?

At the September 2009 meeting of the Joint Commission Executive Briefings, the average turnaround time was reported as two to three days. This means an organization that believes it has an opportunity to clarify findings should begin the clarification process immediately after receipt of its on-site report.

Another change was the format of the survey report. If your organization utilizes The Joint Commission for deemed status, the report has been modified to provide a crosswalk between the noncompliant standards and CMS' *Conditions of Participation (CoP)* with A-tags. This is a great improvement and will help accreditation specialists learn the *CoP*s and how they correlate with the Joint Commission standards. It is about time that the requirements are coming closer together and we don't have to say to staff members, "The Joint Commission requires this and CMS requires that," which makes our credibility go down the drain.

The report will also identify the level of criticality for elements of performance (EP) that are found to be insufficiently compliant. Recall that criticality is defined as follows:

- 2 in a triangle = situational decision rules
- 3 in a triangle = direct impact
- 4 in a triangle = indirect impact

A feature that should be helpful as an internal reminder is the labeling of each EP as to whether the evidence of standards compliance (ESC) is due within 45 days for direct impact or 60 days for indirect impact. Another feature coincides with a new acronym: OCO, which stands for Observed but Corrected On-site. EPs found to be noncompliant but corrected while the surveyors are still on-site will be labeled as OCO.

The Joint Commission report samples are under a copyright and cannot be included in this book. Please see the October 2009 issue of *Perspectives* for a review of the sample reports.

The Next Step: Identifying Opportunities for Clarification

When findings include RFIs, an extranet submission of clarifying ESC or ESC is mandated. Utilizing the report provided at the close of the on-site survey, a prompt evaluation of the findings is warranted to determine whether clarifications are possible for any of the noncompliant standards. Effective January 1, 2009, all clarifications were to be submitted within 10 business days after a final decision report had been posted to the extranet.

> **Field Experience**
>
>
>
> Some clients continue to be reluctant to clarify RFIs, especially if the number is low and they feel many more findings could have been identified. But the problem with holding back on clarification is that it is difficult to correct a process that is not broken! When fixes are attempted for unbroken processes, organizations tend to create "over-requirements" that add complexity but no actual value. There is no harm in attempting a clarification, so if you believe you may be able to do so, give it a try.

Before you begin, review the document titled "Guidelines for Submission of Evidence of Standards Compliance" on the Joint Commission's Web site at *www.jointcommission.org/NR/ rdonlyres/81F83BEB-297C-4AF5-9B8B-DF0AE1583B62/0/Guidelines_ESC_Submissionv15.pdf*. It seems that many clients are not aware of this document, but hidden on page 3 is a section titled "Clarification (optional)." This document provides the information necessary to prepare a clarification, and therefore you can use it to determine whether a clarification is even possible.

How to assess for clarification opportunities

Category A EPs are either present or not present. In a clarification, you must demonstrate that the organization was compliant at the time of survey. This is not easy, but it can be done.

Category A clarification

Let's use PI.02.01.01 EP 8 as an illustration. Say your organization uses the results of data analysis to identify improvement opportunities. If you feel your organization was compliant at the time of survey, because you have examples of how data analysis resulted in findings and correlated actions were then implemented, you must formulate the following for a clarification:

- What policy or procedure was present before the survey that supports the requirement for data analysis to occur following data collection, and as a result of the analysis, actions for improvement are implemented? Perhaps your organization's performance improvement plan or prioritized listing of performance improvement projects could be helpful in this regard.

- Who at the highest level approved the policy? Use names and titles, such as John Smith, CEO.

- When was the policy approved and what was the effective date?

- How were staff members informed about the policy and procedure requirements? Describe the mechanism of disseminating the expectations of data analysis and selection of correlated interventions for improvement.

- Why did the surveyor not have access to the information or why wasn't it provided to the surveyor during the survey? This can get tricky, and you have to state the issue exactly as it happened. For instance, you may have provided documents to the surveyor, but he or she either rushed through them or performed a superficial review and may have drawn premature conclusions that the EP was not met. Avoid any negative comments regarding the surveyor's behavior; adhere to the facts and state exactly what happened.

> **Field Experience**
>
> Prepare this information as a narrative statement using a word processing program, and then cut and paste the content to the extranet for submission to The Joint Commission. This is a big time-saver as word processing outside the extranet is more user-friendly.

A surveyor must identify at least three instances of noncompliance during a survey for a category C EP to be cited. Your job is to demonstrate that with a larger sample size, the organization would be in compliance. If you believe the element in question will likely measure at 90% or greater compliance, promptly determine sample sizes, a method for selecting the sample, and a plan for data collection for category C EPs. You may have to begin collecting data before you receive the final report, as 10 days can pass quickly and will feel even shorter with the final reports being posted more quickly.

Category C clarification

There are two ways to construct a clarification, but the most common is presented first.

Using the sampling criteria in the How to Use This Book chapter in the standards manual, select the minimum number of samples based on your organization's average daily census at the time of the survey. For example, if your organization's average daily census was 352 during the survey, you need to select a sample of 50 cases.

You must choose your sample from a report of patients that were admitted but were discharged 30 days prior to the start of the survey. For example, if your survey began on October 12, count October 11 as day one and count back 30 days.

After running your report of the 30-day population, select your sample by either downloading the report into Excel using the random sample commands, which is beyond the scope of this book, or select every X number of cases calculated by the volume of the report and divide that number by your sample size. Using the preceding example, therefore, you would divide the total number of patients by 50 and then select every Nth patient.

> **Key Concept**
>
> Carefully construct your sample without introducing any bias. A clarification could be rejected if the sampling method is flawed. Do not use the term *random sample*, as that term has many meanings and is often biased since the selection process is haphazard and not structured.

Required categories of data must be collected for the audit. These categories include medical record number, attending physician, number of correct items for the topic, number of incorrect items for the topic, and total number of items. Create a table and use these categories as your column labels. This is how the data will be entered into the extranet at the time of submission.

An alternative method to performing an audit is to utilize data that were already collected as a component of the organization's performance improvement plan or standards compliance assessment. This is not as popular as conducting an audit, because it is difficult to meet the sample requirements and to demonstrate randomization. Also, the data have to match the time frames of immediately prior to the survey; therefore, the data collection would have to have been continuous. I recommend that you reserve this method for situations in which the organization is in an adverse accreditation decision and you must pull out all stops to attempt to clarify noncompliant standards.

Clients frequently ask me, "When will we receive a response from The Joint Commission following our submission of clarifications?" Unfortunately, the answer is "That depends." For example, I assisted a client in submitting clarifications following an issuance of predenial of accreditation, and it was three months before the organization received the response of acceptance.

Upon submission of clarifications, your organization will receive a confirmation of receipt that will be posted on the extranet. I recommend that you work with your account executive to seek information on the status of your clarifications. Should the clarifications be accepted, the EPs will be removed from the report and a new report will be posted to the extranet site. If a clarification is denied, the finding stands as was indicated in the final report, and an ESC will need to be submitted.

Evidence of standards compliance

For each noncompliant EP for which clarification was not attempted or was attempted and was not accepted, you must prepare a submission of how the organization corrected the noncompliance. Be cautious of time frames, remembering that EPs labeled with a "3" inside a triangle have a direct impact on patient care and that an ESC must be submitted within 45 days of the date the final report was posted to the extranet. EPs labeled with a "4" inside a triangle (a new icon initiated in the latter part of 2009) are considered to have an indirect effect on patient care and require an ESC be submitted within 60 days.

> **Key Concept**
>
>
>
> All actions are to be written in past tense; nothing should be entered into the report with a future date, as compliance must be met within the required time frames. When asked to preview a client's draft ESCs, I've noticed that phrases such as *will be implemented, has been scheduled,* or *awaiting arrival* are still being used. These are neon lights to the Joint Commission review committee. When ESC tasks are decentralized, authors need to be carefully oriented to the expected corrections and methods of drafting the submissions. There should be no surprises as the write-ups are collected. When written well, the ESC should tell a story that is precise and in chronological order of occurrence.

The medication management—MM.04.01.01 EP 13, requiring a hospital to implement medication order policies—is an example of an EP with direct impact on patient care. In the example shown in Figure 9.1 in this book's online appendix, the hospital's policy required an indication to be provided with PRN orders, and this was missing in at least three occurrences.

If this EP were found to be noncompliant, an action to initiate this practice might be circulation of the requirement in multiple media types, such as mailers, memos, e-mail blitzes, posters, newsletters, and so forth. Staff members involved in accepting telephone orders would also be reminded of this requirement. Actions should be focused on the failed portion of the policy and should not include other items. A policy revision would not be expected unless the organization wanted to narrow its own requirements or add consequences for not adhering to the policy. The title of the individual approving the correction process would be documented and ready for submission in 45 days.

An example of an indirect EP is PC.01.02.01 EP 1, requiring the hospital to define in writing the scope and content of any screening, assessment, and reassessment information it collects. This is a category A EP with documentation required. Hypothetically, it is likely that the policy would need to be revised. The revision, who approved the revision, who approved the corrective action, how it was implemented, and dates for all would need to be submitted within 60 days.

Measure of success (MOS)

If you come across an EP labeled with a circled "M" when you are preparing ESCs, you must describe at the time of submission the method of measuring the EP after acceptance by The Joint Commission. In such cases, you should think of the saying "I am from Missouri, so show me [that you have really brought this element of performance into compliance]."

You will be formulating a way to quantify your actions to prove that the process is now compliant. During the 2008 cleanup of standards and on into 2009, revisions were being made so that only category C EPs included an MOS. As changes were made, they were published in *Perspectives* and were added to standards manual updates.

MOS data are to be collected for a period of four months following acceptance of the ESC. Utilize the methods of selecting sample sizes and collecting data described for clarifying a category C EP. The only difference is the sampling time period. Compliance is calculated each month, and at the conclusion of four months, the average of the aggregated four months will be calculated as a percentage. To be considered in compliance, a percentage greater than 90% must be achieved. The achieved percentage will be submitted to The Joint Commission via the extranet.

Field Experience

As they formulate their MOS for submission with the ESC, some hospitals provide additional awareness to the folks who are involved in the process that will be measured. Let them know how key it is that their practice matches the actions attested to and that failure to achieve a 90% compliance rate at the end of four months could result in conditonal accreditation.

Immediate threat to health or safety

Should a situation exist that triggers a determination of immediate threat to health or safety, an expedited decision of preliminary denial of accreditation may be issued and the organization has up to 72 hours to eliminate the threat; if more time is warranted, interim safety measures must be implemented and up to 23 days will be allowed for complete resolution.

Once the organization notifies The Joint Commission that it has resolved the immediate threat, The Joint Commission will conduct an "abatement" survey to validate that the threat has been corrected. Then, the preliminary denial of accreditation will be changed to a conditional accreditation and that status will remain until a follow-up survey is conducted to ensure that the correction has been sustained.

An organization may appeal an accreditation decision by contacting The Joint Commission within five days of confirmation of a preliminary denial of accreditation. Readers should reference the "Review and Appeal Procedures" section in the standards manual for more information.

Situational decisions

Situational decision rules are rules listed in the Accreditation Process chapter of the standards manual. Enactment of a rule could result in preliminary denial of accreditation or conditional accreditation. In this adverse situation, all ESCs must be submitted within 45 days and a validation survey will be conducted to evaluate implementation of corrective action.

> **Key Concept**
>
>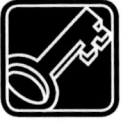
>
> Validation surveys are specific to the adverse finding, and in that regard an organization should carefully construct its ESC submissions. Ensure that the "fixes" are accurate and true in all areas of operation. Adverse accreditation decisions should be taken very seriously. When in doubt about how to proceed, contract with a consulting firm that has a documented track record of managing RFIs and adverse accreditation decisions. Remember, your participation in Medicare and Medicaid programs is at risk.

After-Survey Activities

After an organization submits its ESCs, the Joint Commission's central office will review the material, and if actions have been taken to address the RFIs, the organization's accreditation decision will be changed to accredited.

If an ESC submission is not accepted, the EP score will remain the same as it was at the conclusion of the survey. If one or more of the standards remain noncompliant, the organization's accreditation decision will become provisional, and a second ESC will be requested for submission within 30 days. If the ESCs are accepted, the organization will be provisional until the MOS results are received. A second rejecton of ESCs will yield an accreditation decision of conditional. Consult the Accreditation Process chapter of your accreditation manual for additional information.

Evaluating the Success of the Organization's Unannounced Survey Plan

Treat the completion of your unannounced survey as a performance improvement outcome and assess the strengths and weaknesses of your unannounced survey readiness plan. You should do this in two separate sessions: one in which you conduct a debriefing of the implementation of the plan, and a second subsequent session in which you discuss the findings related to noncompliant standards.

This first session is not an exercise to discuss perceptions of surveyor accuracy, RFI clarifications, or how to submit ESCs; it is a retrospective review of your organization's methods of preparing for an unannounced survey.

Include the following people in your debriefing of the plan:
- Accreditation specialist
- Designated staff members with assigned tasks during the survey

The following are suggested work steps for the debriefing:
- List the steps of the unannounced plan that worked well and achieved the desired results
- List identified issues or concerns and determine what processes in the defined plan did not occur as anticipated
- Seek input from attendees regarding alternative methods to prevent a reoccurrence

- Revise the unannounced plan and test it in a subsequent drill after all clarifications, ESCs, and MOSs are completed

Include these people in your second session to discuss the findings of noncompliant standards:

- Chapter team leaders or leaders of special issues, depending on your chosen approach to standards compliance
- Accreditation specialist

Perform the following:

- Review the survey report
- Discuss which findings were anticipated or unanticipated based on your internal assessment, presurvey tracers, or data monitoring
- Identify factors that may have affected results
- Brainstorm alternative methods of promoting continuous standards compliance

Maintain Survey Readiness

Now that your survey is completed, your work has just begun. You must keep the momentum going and stay focused on continually meeting the Joint Commission requirements. Other forces will vie for attention, such as changes in personnel, the introduction of new services, building renovations, and other competing initiatives, and you play a key role in helping to prevent Joint Commission compliance from being pushed to the back burner.

Stay current with standard and survey changes

As the accreditation specialist, you are challenged to ensure that you maintain your expertise by staying current with changes. This task is an onerous job in itself. The following is a suggested approach:

- Make certain that you maintain the *Comprehensive Accreditation Manual for Hospitals* or the *Comprehensive Accreditation Manual for Critical Access Hospitals* as well as any other manuals you might need for other accreditation programs such as home care, long-term care, laboratory, behavioral healthcare, or ambulatory care. Manual updates previously arrived in June 2009, and will be issued again in late 2009, according to the October issue of *Perspectives.*

Ensure timely receipt of the *Perspectives* publication. Scan the "Contents" outline to identify potentially hot topics for your organization. Distribute a copy of any pertinent article to individuals involved in the specific topic. Save paper and don't send a copy to every department director. They do not have the drive to read this type of periodical; their priority is the function of the department for which they are accountable. So, face reality and spoon-feed the appropriate articles to the appropriate people.

- Subscribe to HCPro's **Briefings on the Joint Commission.** This non–Joint Commission publication is chock-full of innovative ideas implemented by others like you, provides you with a large group of individuals with whom to network, and alerts you to changes that you may have overlooked in other publications.

- Sign up for an RSS feed of "What's New" on the Joint Commission Web site *(www.jointcommission.org/NewsRoom/rss.htm)*.

- Bookmark the site for the Joint Commission's FAQs that now includes the National Patient Safety Goals and standards. Set a task on your electronic calendar to remind you to check the FAQs monthly for any new postings. Effective dates are listed so that you can determine what is new since your last visit to the site. Build your standards interpretation skills by reading the question and coming up with a possible answer before you read the one provided by the Standards Interpretation Group.

- Bookmark the Joint Commission's extranet site. Determine how frequently you should enter this site to watch for e-mails, updates, and general information. Many of the Joint Commission's communications are being posted to the extranet and are not being sent via another e-mail site or hard-copy mailing.

Identify Methods to Monitor Standards Compliance

Monitor your organization's Strategic Surveillance System (S3) score. Consider adding this score to your organization's performance dashboard.

If you are unfamiliar with the S3 score, explore the user guide and tutorial found on the extranet. Quarterly as the score is posted, evaluate your hospital's performance in relationship to the 14 priority focus areas. The S3 data are also sorted by clinical service groups (CSG). Hospital CSGs are derived from CMS-defined classifications of data that roll up into diagnosis-related group data. CMS collects Medicare Provider Analysis and Review (MedPAR) data and includes more than 800 data elements from short stays and inpatient hospital stays. Your S3 score contains the most current three years' worth of MedPAR data available from CMS regarding indicators for complications, mortality, and average length of stay. As I stated in Chapter 1, The Joint Commission is discussing possible removal of MedPAR data due to the lag time in receiving the data.

In the July 2009 issue of *Perspectives,* planned enhancements to S3 scores were announced. A "What's New" report will detail changes specific to your hospital that had occurred subsequent to the last quarterly update of the S3 score. As new data are added, such as Hospital Consumer Assessment of Healthcare Providers and Systems data, this information will be included in the report. A trended report is provided that displays the hospital's S3 score over time. This would be an excellent report to share with organizational leaders.

Conduct internal tracers

Conduct patient tracers to evaluate compliance with the organization's policies and procedures. Chapter 5 discussed the use of tracers as a follow-up to the internal assessment; tracers should also be used following actual surveys. The appendix at the back of this book includes a "Show Me" tracer (Appendix A.2) generously shared by Altru Health System, and additional tracer formats are supplied in the appendix of this book (Appendices A.8-A.12), so you can customize them to your policy requirements. Coordinate this activity by establishing a schedule of patient care units and perform tracers at a volume that seems appropriate for your organization. The tracer forms should be dynamic; delete items as continuous compliance is achieved, and add new items as changes in standards occur or noncompliance is identified from another source.

> **Key Concept**
>
>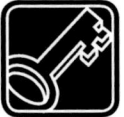
>
> Use staff members from other departments to conduct tracers. Not only does this provide a new set of eyes, but it also increases appreciation of the complexity of the patient care delivery system in patient care areas. Consider having a team of two different disciplines: a nurse (from an area other than the one being traced) and a pharmacist. Don't forget to include your administrative staff.

Involve the unit clerks in tracers as well. They are instrumental in assembling and filing various components of the medical record, and an organized medical record is the first step toward a successful tracer. Let them know how valuable they are in relocating misfiled documents, alerting staff members to forms that are missing signatures, ensuring that patient identification is contained on each page within the record, and ensuring that the record tabs are in consistent order.

Work closely with the performance improvement staff

Often, performance improvement data are generated from other sources, such as the hospital's performance improvement program, but are not shared with the accreditation specialist. Connect with your performance improvement director and discuss the types of data that could assist the organization in monitoring standards compliance. If an inventory of data collection is available, request to be copied on results.

Maintain an ongoing action plan

In Chapter 4, we discussed the benefits of conducting a thorough and accurate internal assessment. Standards scored as noncompliant should be immediately moved to the organization's action plan for monitoring until compliance is achieved.

The Standards Compliance Action Plan should be dynamic and be the basis for leadership to know at any time how compliant the organization is with the Joint Commission standards. Realistic time frames for corrective action should be documented, with an individual accountable for each step.

Update leaders on your progress

Whether you have a committee in charge of oversight or whether the hospital leadership functions as this body, keep leaders continually updated on your organization's progress. Remember that the philosophy is not to have any surprises. You must communicate issues of noncompliance that are not being resolved. If you know of problems and you do not pass such items up the chain of command, you become part of the problem. Be prepared to answer questions from leadership regarding the likelihood that the noncompliant issues will be identified in an actual survey if they are not corrected.

Establish a positive relationship with your Joint Commission account executive

Consider this individual to be your door into The Joint Commission. The October 2009 issue of *Perspectives* discussed the improved customer service initiatives that have been undertaken in the past year. Authors announced the teaming of account executives with program-specific standards interpretation professionals, and increased education of account executives regarding the accreditation process. Consult with your account representative and maintain notes of these conversations.

Ask for assistance when communications from The Joint Commission are not clear or understandable. If you do not receive a level of service that is expected, contact The Joint Commission and ask to speak to the supervisor of the account executives. Should you reach a dead end, never hesitate to search out Ann Scott Blouin, executive vice president of Accreditation and Certification Operations. Repeatedly at the Briefings, she voiced the need to improve customer service and your feedback was encouraged.

Build your resource library

You can purchase from HCPro a bound version of the updated *CoPs*, titled *The CMS Interpretive Guidelines for the Hospital Conditions of Participation-Updated*. Go to *www.hcmarketplace.com/ prod-6613.html* for more information.

Because The Joint Commission serves as the deemed status for CMS, you might find the following Web site helpful: *http://tinyurl.com/yda8pah*. On this Web site, releases are listed in reverse order, with the most recent release located at the bottom of the spreadsheet, so don't give up before you scroll downward.

Obtain a copy of your state health department's regulation for hospitals and other healthcare organizations. When an EP references "other state laws and regulations," this would be a probable source of information.

Encourage your human resources department to maintain references to licensed practitioners' scope of practice within your state. With the development of preprinted order sets, protocols, and guidelines, scopes of practice are invaluable references.

Conferences and networking

Conferences on accreditation readiness are available through HCPro, Inc., Joint Commission Resources, Inc., and other entities. Consider participating in audio conferences, which include a wealth of information without the cost of travel. Conferences are essential for gaining experience in accurately interpreting accreditation standards and troubleshooting areas of noncompliance.

Consider joining a related e-mail chat group, such as HCPro's Accreditation Talk or Patient Safety Talk listservs, to communicate with your peers regarding standards interpretation, survey readiness ideas, and information about the Joint Commission surveyors.

Join the Association for Healthcare Accreditation Professionals (AHAP), a membership association started in 2006. AHAP is a vibrant community of accreditation professionals who share challenges, knowledge, and experiences. It offers its members staff training ideas, tips on professional development, and educational information for accreditation. Members receive the much-needed opportunity to network with accreditation peers through member publications, task forces, quarterly live chats with peers via teleconference, and an annual conference. Visit *www.accreditationprofessional.org* for more information.

RFI-proof your policies and procedures

> **Key Concept**
>
>
>
> Before finalizing a policy or procedure, compare its content to the Joint Commission requirements, CMS requirements, and state regulations. Determine whether the medical staff bylaws/rules and regulations have addressed the topic, and make sure none of the documents offer conflicting information. Because many RFIs are based on staff members not following their own organization's policies, research what is minimally required by each regulatory entity and encourage leadership not to raise the bar of expectation to a level that cannot be achieved.

Assess orientation programs

Assess hospital orientation programs to ensure that revised practices and accreditation requirements are being incorporated into the curriculum. Take a look at your hospital's training needs—from physicians to the frontline staff—drawing upon the advice of your education staff members. Consider whether the staff needs knowledge-based training (e.g., refreshers on fire-drill instructions or confidentiality policies) or survey process training (e.g., a description of what to expect during unit tours).

Understand line management responsibilities

Don't confuse standards compliance with poor performance of job responsibilities. The accreditation specialist does not have authority over personnel and their failure to follow policies and procedures. The Joint Commission steering committee or a similar oversight body for accreditation readiness should not be involved in performance issues after education has been provided to the staff. For example, failure to complete a dietary assessment within the defined time frame must be addressed by the manager, not the accreditation specialist.

TEST YOUR KNOWLEDGE

1. True or false: Once The Joint Commission issues a preliminary denial of accreditation following the finding of a threat to health and safety, the decision is final and appeals are not accepted.

Answer: False. An organization may inform The Joint Commission of its intent to appeal within five days of confirmation of the accreditation decision.

2. When formulating an evidence of standards compliance for a category A element of performance, which of the following items should be included?
    A. Title of individual who approved the revised policy
    B. Date the policy was approved
    C. Newsletter article to be published at a later date
    D. Description of how employees were informed of changes

    1. A, B, C
    2. A, C, D
    3. A, B, D
    4. All of the above

Answer: 3. All activities must have been completed by the time the ESC is submitted. An article for a newsletter yet to be published is unacceptable.

3. Which of the following are true regarding a measure of success?
    A. Multiple MOS attempts to achieve compliance are allowed
    B. Unbiased sampling methods are required
    C. An average of four months' worth of data collection will be submitted
    D. A score of 90% or greater equals compliance

    1. A, B, C
    2. B, C, D
    3. A, C, D
    4. All of the above

Answer: 2. Conditional accreditation will be recommended if the organization fails to clear noncompliant standards after two opportunities to do so.

APPENDIX

Additional Forms

The following tools have been referenced throughout this book and have been included here for your reference.

All of the items included in this appendix, including samples mentioned in the text, as well as any charts or graphics located in the body of this book are also available online at: *www.hcpro.com/ downloads/8088*. This library also contains numerous additional tools for download not included in the print version, so please take the opportunity to check out all of the bonus materials included on the web page.

Figure A.1 ■ "Show Me" Tracer—Most Challenging Standards

SHOW ME

Date: _____   Staff Assisting Tracer Team _____
Reviewer(s) 1. _____   2. _____

% that JC NPSGs and Standards were identified as "not compliant" in 2008 during JC surveys in our nation.

TOPIC	FINDINGS: check items indicating compliance	Describe Non-compliance Issues	Staff Name(s) for Follow-up
Do Not Use Abbreviations Is there a poster in the department? Yes No SHOW ME Some examples are listed in the next box. Review these with the staff.	Most often used incorrectly: ☐ 1. U = write unit ☐ 2. QD, QOD = write daily or every other day ☐ 3. Trailing zero = never write a zero by itself after a decimal point (X mg) ☐ 4. Lack of leading zero = Always use a zero before a decimal point (0.X mg) ☐ 5. MSO4, MS, MgSO4 = write "morphine sulfate" or "magnesium sulfate" ☐ 6. Nitro drip = write "nitroglycerin drip" or "Nipride drip" ☐ 7. Inform staff that we (Altru) audit for compliance with "do not use abbreviations" via the pharmacy POMS system 2-4 times per year or more if compliance declines. NONCOMPLIANCE CITED 18 % OF THE TIME		
Timeliness of reporting and receipt of critical test / results / values	☐ 1. How much time is allowed to report the test results to the provider once the result is known? _____ (60 minutes) ☐ 2. What tests are identified as critical tests for Altru Health System: Policy #2126 #1. Stat CT for the Brain for Stroke, ordered by ER Reporting time = Report in 2 hours #2. Stat Echocardiogram Reporting time = Report in 90 minutes #3. Stat In-patient Blood Gases by RT Reporting time = Report in 60 minutes #4. Stat Troponin ordered inpatient in ICU or SCCU Reporting time = Report in 120 minutes ☐ 3. Staff write down or enter the order or test result into the computer, read back the complete order or test result, and the individual who gave the order confirms the information. ☐ 4. Data regarding the timeliness of reporting information to the provider is collected and reported to the Patient Safety Committee. NONC0MPLIANCE CITED 41 % OF THE TIME		
Medication Reconciliation (a process for comparing the patient's current meds with those ordered for the patient) SHOW ME Review a current patient record.	What is the process for Medication Reconciliation? 1. A list of medications is created upon admission or entry to the inpatient or the outpatient setting 100 % of the time. *CHECK A CHART FOR THE PRESCENCE OF THE ADMIT MRR (Home Medication List). Admit MRR is present? MR#_____ ☐ Yes ☐ No 2. This list is communicated to the provider ☐ Yes ☐ No		

L/Janelle Holth/Tracers/2009 Tracers/Challenging Standards 8-09   Page 1 of 4

Figure A.1 ■ "Show Me" Tracer—Most Challenging Standards (Cont.)

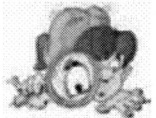
SHOW ME

TOPIC	FINDINGS: check items indicating compliance	Describe Non-compliance Issues	Staff Name(s) for Follow-up
	3. The list is transferred with the patient as they travel through the health system ☐ Yes ☐ No 4. A complete list is sent home with the patient upon discharge. ☐ Yes ☐ No NONCOMPLIANCE CITED 22 % OF THE TIME		
Label all medications / solutions on and off the field. SHOW ME Observe a procedure (if at all possible.)	What steps are involved with labeling medications? 1. Whenever something is not immediately administered, it is labeled. ☐ Yes ☐ No 2. No batch labeling ☐ Yes ☐ No 3. No batch filling ☐ Yes ☐ No 4. Explain the components that are to be on the label. ☐ a. Name of medication ☐ b. Strength ☐ c. Amount if not apparent by viewing the container CITED 18 % OF THE TIME		
Labeling SHOW ME Observe a procedure.	LABELING OF MEDICATIONS: 1. Are their procedures done at the bedside on this unit? ☐ Yes ☐ No 2. Are their any times that you take a medication from its original container without immediately administering it? ☐ Yes ☐ No ☐ IF yes, how do you label these medications: _____ 3. Are specimens labeling at the bedside or in the presence of the patient? ☐ Yes ☐ No		
The administration of moderate sedation, deep sedation or anesthesia is planned. SHOW ME	Review documentation for deep or moderate sedation. 1. Components of the sedation form are complete. MR#_____ ☐ pre-anesthesia assessment completed (gold) ☐ ASA score ☐ past anesthesia history ☐ lung assessment ☐ cardiac assessment ☐ airway assessment of class, neck, and teeth ☐ anesthesia plan ☐ risks, benefits and alternatives discussed with patient/family NONCOMPLIANCE CITED 17 % OF THE TIME		
Operative or other procedures are planned SHOW ME	☐ informed consent obtained by physician with physician signature on surgical permit. MR #_____ ☐ Date next to physician signature ☐ Time next to physician signature ☐ permit dated by patient signature ☐ permit timed by patient signature ☐ Informed consent is dated and timed before the authorization is dated and times NONCOMPLIANCE CITED 17 % OF THE TIME		

L/Janelle Holth/Tracers/2009 Tracers/Challenging Standards 8-09   Page 2 of 4

Appendix

Figure A.1 ■ "Show Me" Tracer—Most Challenging Standards (Cont.)

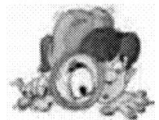
SHOW ME

TOPIC	FINDINGS: check items indicating compliance	Describe Non-compliance Issues	Staff Name(s) for Follow-up
Medications are properly and safely stored. Medications are safe and secure at all times. SHOW ME	**STORAGE:** **Tracer team members - Check the medication refrigerator.** ☐ Temperature log is complete. ☐ Verbalizes who monitors the temperature? ☐ No past due meds are in the refrigerator. ☐ Verbalizes process for returning medications to pharmacy? ☐ No medications are left unattended in the nurse's station. ☐ Observe alcoves - No medications are left unattended on the counter tops ☐ Observe alcoves – Medication drawers are locked CITED 34 % OF THE TIME		
Two Patient Identifiers SHOW ME **Observe 1 or more of the following:** 1. medication admin 2. Hanging IV fluids 3. Beginning blood admin 4. Delivery of PT, OT, Speech, RT, SW or dietary services. (any care, treatment or service to the patient begins with performing 2 identifiers)	☐ full name (is always the 1st identifier) ☐ date of birth ☐ MRUN (one of the above will be the 2nd identifier depending on the service provided) ☐ Administering medication ☐ Collecting blood samples and other specimens for clinical testing ☐ Providing other treatments or procedures ☐ Containers used for blood and other specimens are labeled in the presence of the patient. We cannot pre-label containers, syringes, or blood tubes. ☐ What is the process if the patient does not have an armband? ☐ What do we do if the patient cannot be involved during patient identification process?		
Hand washing SHOW ME 1. **Observe a procedure** 2. **Observe any delivery of care, treatment or services to the patient.** **Provide immediate feedback.** Staff / title observed: _____ _____	☐ Hands washed with soap and water when visibly soiled or contaminated ☐ Entering and leaving patient room ☐ Before and after gloving ☐ Before a procedure **Hand antisepsis after the following:** ☐ Contact with a patient's intact skin (taking a pulse or B/P) ☐ Contact with blood or body fluids ☐ Contact with inanimate objects in the immediate vicinity of the patient (equipment) ☐ Before donning sterile gloves ☐ Apply 3-5 ml of soap to hands ☐ Rub hands together vigorously for 15 seconds ☐ Avagard D, use 1 pumpful or ☐ Alcare, use a palmful of foam		

L/Janelle Holth/Tracers/2009 Tracers/Challenging Standards 8-09   Page 3 of 4

Figure A.1 ■ "Show Me" Tracer—Most Challenging Standards (Cont.)

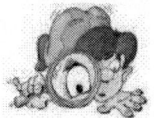
SHOW ME

TOPIC	FINDINGS: check items indicating compliance	Describe Non-compliance Issues	Staff Name(s) for Follow-up
Patient Involvement in their care SHOW ME Interview a patient / family	Are staff using 2 identifiers before delivery of care, treatment or services? ☐ Yes ☐ No Discussion with:_____ Room #_____, MR #_____		
Patient Involvement in their care SHOW ME Interview a patient / family	What 3 items do we need to educate our patient about? ☐ 1. Hand Hygiene ☐ 2. Respiratory Hygiene ☐ 3. Contact Isolation ☐ What tool do we use to provide education to patients on the above 3 items:_____ (blue Patient Education Safety booklet)		
Employee / Patient Safety	1. If you had a concern about employee/patient safety that is not being addressed by our Health Organization you can notify JC without retaliation. True_____ False_____ Where do you find out how to contact JC? a. Patient Relations Brochure b. Policy #2513 Altru Corporate Compliance		
Blanket Warmer SHOW ME	☐ Blanket warmer (s) temperature is set to not exceed 110 degrees. ☐ N/A Temperature reading on the blanket warmer ___ degrees		
INFORMATION	**FOR STAFF**		

1. Noncompliance Cited during 46% of the 2008 surveys for:	**Environment of Care:** Newly constructed and existing environments are designed and maintained to comply with the Life Safety Code.
	Surveyors may ask questions about the following:
	    1. Hallways being clear for ease access and transport of patients
	    2. Staff knowledge of what to do if a fire occurs
	    3. How are patients evacuated?
	    4. What are some safety processes with the use of oxygen?		

L/Janelle Holth/Tracers/2009 Tracers/Challenging Standards 8-09   Page 4 of 4

Figure A.2 — Labeling of Secondary Containers

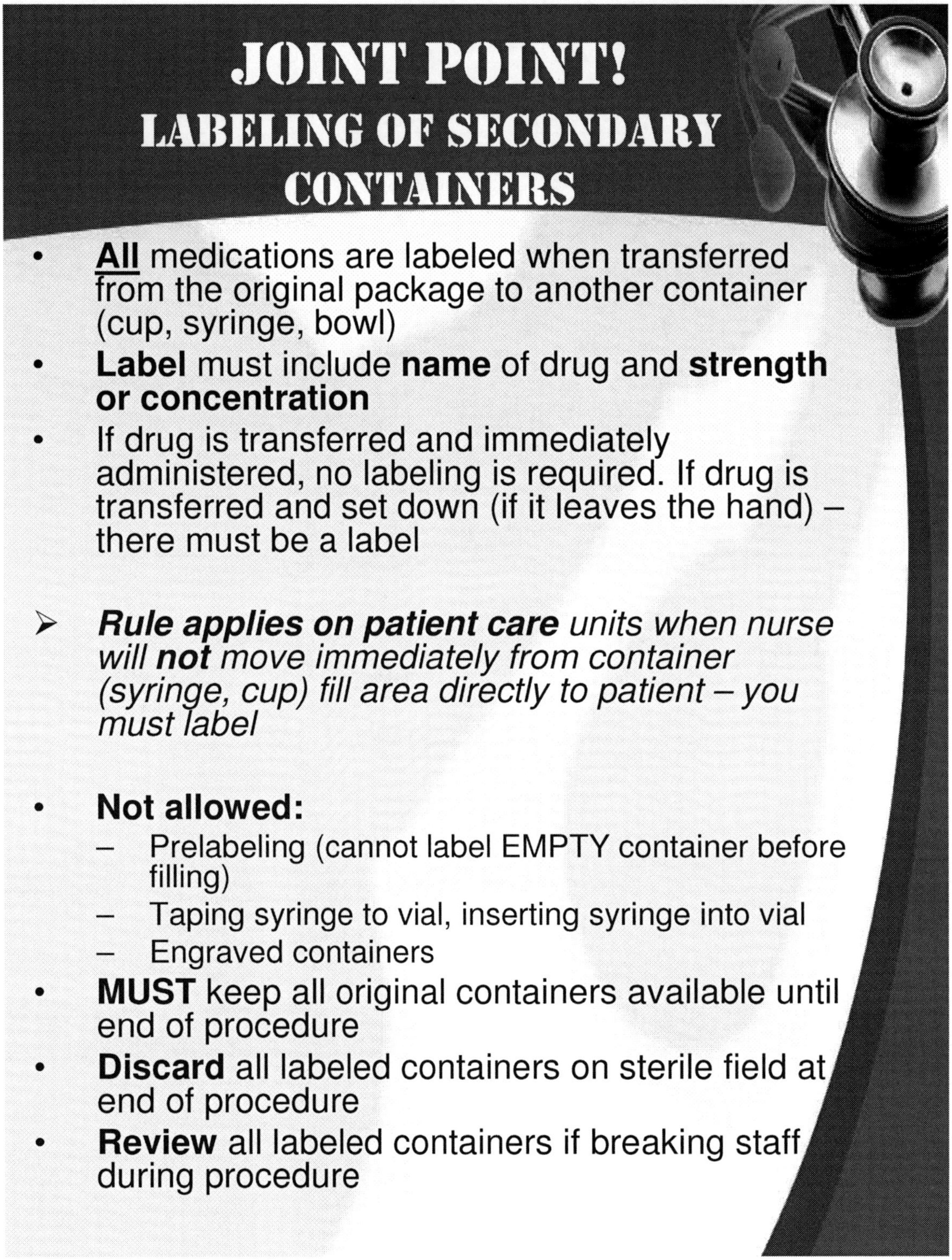

JOINT POINT!
LABELING OF SECONDARY CONTAINERS

- **All** medications are labeled when transferred from the original package to another container (cup, syringe, bowl)
- **Label** must include **name** of drug and **strength or concentration**
- If drug is transferred and immediately administered, no labeling is required. If drug is transferred and set down (if it leaves the hand) – there must be a label

> *Rule applies on patient care* units when nurse will **not** move immediately from container (syringe, cup) fill area directly to patient – you must label

- **Not allowed:**
  - Prelabeling (cannot label EMPTY container before filling)
  - Taping syringe to vial, inserting syringe into vial
  - Engraved containers
- **MUST** keep all original containers available until end of procedure
- **Discard** all labeled containers on sterile field at end of procedure
- **Review** all labeled containers if breaking staff during procedure

Figure A.3 — Improving Patient Identification

JOINT POINT!
TWO (2) IDENTIFIERS

Improve the accuracy of patient identification

- Use two patient identifiers (patient name, date of birth, or when necessary medical record number; **never** the room number or physical location) with the participation of the patient.

 Stop using the patient's room number in conversation, **particularly** at the nurse's station, use the patient's *NAME*

What does with <u>participation of the patient</u> mean?

- When you are providing care, treatment or services that involve more than minimal risk to the patient, you should obtain patient involvement (some type of agreement by patient with identifiers)

    - **If the patient is unreliable (unable to communicate, confused, etc.)** family members or the patient's nurse should be the responsible caregiver designated to verify identity

- Label containers used for blood and other specimens in the presence of the patient

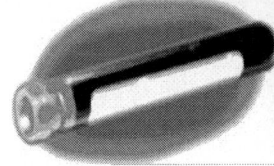

Figure A.4 — Patient Reporting of Safety Concerns

JOINT POINT!
HOW PATIENTS REPORT SAFETY CONCERNS

- **Staff is to encourage patients to report any quality of care or safety concerns**
  - Concerns should be reported to the patient's nurse
  - If nurse cannot resolve, concern is brought to the supervisor
  - Patient can also report to the Patient Advocate ext: 1234
  - If not satisfied patient can report to The Joint Commission
    1-800-944-6610
  - ❖ Staff is to educate patients and their families that <<hospital>> **encourages** this reporting

Figure A.5 — Guidelines for Surgical/Procedural Documentation Requirements

ABC Health System
Guidelines for Surgical/Procedural Documentation Requirements

Revised February 02, 2009

This is not an all-inclusive list of procedures but is intended to serve as a guideline for minimum documentation requirement for elective procedures.

Definitions:
- **Operative Procedures**: any procedure performed within the OR suite; includes cesarean sections performed in OB
- **High-risk procedures**: A procedure that may or may not be an invasive procedure but places the patient at considerable physiological risk and has increased potential for adverse outcomes. Occurrences of adverse events or complications would not be considered unusual.
- **Moderate-risk procedures**: A procedure involving puncture or incision of the skin or insertion of an instrument or foreign material into the body that puts the patient at a lower risk of physiological or adverse outcome. Adverse events or complications would be unusual.
- **Low-risk procedures**: Non-invasive or invasive procedure with minimal risk for physiological or adverse outcomes. Adverse events or complications would be rare.

- Expectations are to follow most stringent guideline i.e., Use of anesthesia with any procedural

Procedure	H & P Type	Practitioner Informed Consent Needed	Universal protocol to be implemented	"Purple Sheet" or 8 elements Post procedure/ surgical NOTE expected	Post Procedural REPORT expected
Procedures in Operating Room:					
All Surgical Procedures	F	Y	I, T; S as applicable	Y	Y
High Risk Procedures Outside Operating Room:					
All General Anesthetics	F	Y	I, T	N/A	Y
Angiography with intervention	F	Y	I, T	Y	Y
Int. Radiology procedures:					
-Kyphoplasty	F	Y	I, S, T	Y	Y
-Radiofrequency ablation	F	Y	I, S, T	Y	Y
-TIPS	F	Y	I, T	Y	Y
-Thrombolysis	F	Y	I, T	Y	Y
Pericardiocentesis	F	Y	I, T	Y	Y

* Brief History and physical if moderate sedation used.
Universal protocol key: I = patient identification S = site marking T = time out
History and physicals: F = full B = brief N/A = not required
Y = yes N = no
LJC/Guidelines for Surgical&Procedural Documentation / Documentation Guidelines for Procedures

Reviewed by: Risk Management, HIM, QM

Approved by Medical Executive Committee: *Date*

Figure A.5 — Guidelines for Surgical/Procedural Documentation Requirements (Cont.)

ABC Health System
Guidelines for Surgical/Procedural Documentation Requirements

Revised February 02, 2009

Procedure	H & P Type	Practitioner-Documented Informed Consent Needed	Universal protocol to be implemented	8 elements Post procedure/surgical NOTE expected	Post Procedural REPORT expected
Moderate Risk Procedures Outside of the Operating Room:					
Monitored Anes Care (MAC), all	B	Y	I,T	N	Y
Moderate Sedation–*any use*	B	Y	I,T	N	Y
Amniocentesis	B	Y	I,T	N	Y
Blood Transfusion	N/A	Y	I	N	N
Bronchoscopy	B	Y	I,T	Y	Y
Cardioversion	B	Y	I,T	N	Y
CRRT	F	Y	I	N	N
CT Guided Biopsy	N/A	Y	I,S,T	Y	Y
Central line/Port insertion / replacement	N/A	Y	I,T	N	Y
Chest tube insertion	N/A	Y	I,S,T	Y	Y
Colonoscopy	B	Y	I,T	Y	Y
Continuous labor epidural	B	Y	I,T	N	Y
Cystoscopy	N/A*	Y	I,T	N	Y
ECT	B	Y (Annual)	I,T	N	Y
EGD	B	Y	I,T	Y	Y
Epidural blood patch	N/A	Y	I,T	N	Y
ERCP	B	Y	I,T	Y	Y
Gastro-jejunosostomy tube placement/replacement	N/A*	Y	I,T	N	Y
Intrathecal injections	N/A	Y	I,T	N	Y
Laser therapy (e.g. veins, liver tumor, eyes)	B	Y	I,S,T	Y	Y
LEEP	N/A*	Y	I,T	N	Y
Lumbar puncture	B	Y	I,T	N	Y
Myelogram	B	Y	I,T	N	Y
NB circumcision	N/A	Y	I,T	Y	Y

* Brief History and physical if moderate sedation used.
Universal protocol key: I = patient identification S = site marking T = time out
History and physicals: F = full B = brief N/A = not required
Y = yes N = no
LJC/Guidelines for Surgical&Procedural Documentation / Documentation Guidelines for Procedures

Reviewed by: Risk Management, HIM, QM

Approved by Medical Executive Committee: *Date*

Figure A.5 — Guidelines for Surgical/Procedural Documentation Requirements (Cont.)

ABC Health System
Guidelines for Surgical/Procedural Documentation Requirements

Revised February 02, 2009

Procedure	H & P Type	Practitioner-Documented Informed Consent Needed	Universal protocol to be implemented	"Purple Sheet" or 8 elements Post procedure/surgical NOTE expected	Post Procedural REPORT expected
Needle localization of breast lesion	N/A	Y	I, S, T	N	Y
Paracentesis	N/A	Y (annual)	I, T	N	Y
Port placement	N/A	Y	I, T	N	Y
Radiation therapy	N/A	Y	I, T	N	Y
Reduction of displaced joints	N/A	Y	I, T	N	Y
Renal dialysis shunt placement	N/A	Y	I, T	N	Y
Stereotactics	N/A	Y	I, S, T	N	Y
TEE	N/A*	Y	I, T	N	Y
Thoracentesis	N/A	Y(annual)	I, S, T	N	Y
Vasectomy	N/A	Y	I, T	N	Y
Low Risk Procedures:					**Brief REPORT/ Progress Note expected**
Acupuncture	N/A	Y	I	N	Y
Cardiac stress test	N/A	N	I	N	Y
Colposcopy	N/A	N	I	N	Y
Cosmetic procedures	N/A	Y	I	N	Y
Joint aspiration / injection	N/A	N	I	N	Y
Nasogastric tube placement	N/A	N	I	N	Y
Phototherapy for bilirubin	N/A	N	I	N	Y
PICC line insertion	N/A	N	I T	N	Y
Removal of small (<2cm) skin lesion	N/A	N	I	N	Y
Renal dialysis, chronic	N/A	Y (Initial)	I	N	Y (Weekly)
Sigmoidoscopy	N/A	Y	I,T	N	Y
Transthoracic Echocardiogram	N/A	N	I	N	Y
Urodynamics	N/A	N	I	N	Y
Uroflow	N/A	N	I	N	Y

* Brief History and physical if moderate sedation used.
Universal protocol key: I = patient identification S = site marking T = time out
History and physicals: F = full B = brief N/A = not required
Y = yes N = no
L:JC/Guidelines for Surgical&Procedural Documentation / Documentation Guidelines for Procedures

3

Reviewed by: Risk Management, HIM, QM

Approved by Medical Executive Committee: *Date*

Appendix

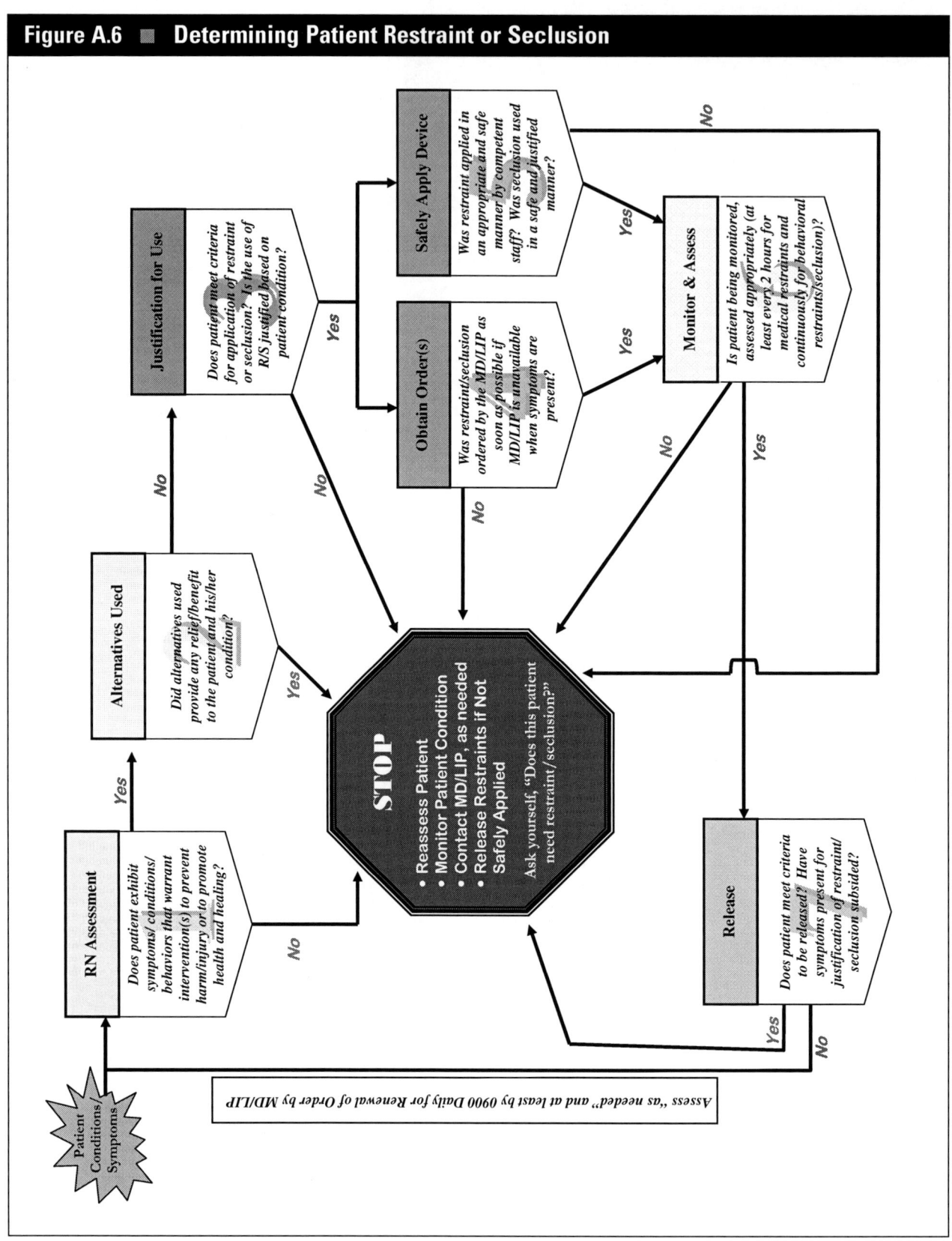

Figure A.6 ■ Determining Patient Restraint or Seclusion

Additional Forms

Figure A.7 ■ Joint Commission Survey Individual Tracer Unit Survey Sheet

Unit: _____

Date of Visit: _____

Place Patient Identification Sticker Here

_____
Name of Patient

_____
Medical Record Number

_____
Date of Admission

Primary Diagnosis:

Male or Female   Age: ____

Secondary Diagnoses:

Special Issues with Patient: (i.e., dialysis, chemotherapy, postoperative pt, infections)

Specific Issues Under Review: (what is the surveyor looking for/at or discussing)

Surveyor Findings: (what did the surveyor say was good or not good)

Surveyor Comments (quotes are always helpful):

Individuals Interviewed (include all)

Any Issues or special comments from Individuals Interviewed

Figure A.8 ■ OB Vaginal Delivery—Tracer Recording Form

Med Record # _____

Reviewer(s) _____ Date _____

TOPIC	FINDINGS: check items indicating compliance	Describe Non-compliance Issues	Staff Name(s) for Follow-up
OB Triage Assessment ☐ N/A	☐ fill in required components ☐ ☐ ☐ ☐		
Pre-delivery Physician Orders	☐ orders obtained prior to initiating IV, labs, etc. ☐ pre-printed orders are initiated by an order ☐ orders are signed, dated and timed		
Inpatient Nursing Assessment	☐ completed within __ hours of admission ☐ home medications list compiled ☐ nutritional screen ☐ functional screen ☐ abuse or neglect screen ☐ discharge planning needs ☐ pain assessment ☐ pain scale ☐ falls risk assessment ☐ cultural/religious issue that affect care ☐ height and weight recorded		
Referrals Triggered from Assessment ☐ N/A	☐ case management ☐ social work		
Labor Education ☐ N/A	☐ education documented		
Labor Progress	☐ documentation entered at appropriate intervals ☐ physician contacted timely as warranted by fetal monitoring ☐ add other requirements ☐		
Pre-epidural Anesthesia Assessment ☐ N/A	☐ pre-anesthesia assessment present ☐ past anesthesia history ☐ heart and lung assessment ☐ informed consent obtained by anesthesia staff		
Immediate Post-delivery Care ☐ N/A	☐ pain assessment conducted ☐ vital signs recorded at required frequency ☐ add other requirements specific to delivery		
Physician's Immediate Post-delivery Note ☐ N/A	☐ handwritten on chart ☐ includes: physician, assistants, description of delivery, neonatal wt. and length, EBL, specimens obtained and patient status		
Postpartum Vital Signs ☐ N/A	☐ every 15 minutes X 4 ☐ every 30 minutes X 2 ☐ every hour X 2		

Page 1 of 2   CONFIDENTIAL

Figure A.8 ■ OB Vaginal Delivery—Tracer Recording Form (Cont.)

TOPIC	FINDINGS: check items indicating compliance	Describe Non-compliance Issues	Staff Name(s) for Follow-up
	☐ once a shift or more frequently if ordered Amend to match hospital policy		
H & P inpatient admission	☐ prenatal records present ☐ update documented within 24 hours of admission ☐ if no prenatal, H & P on record within 24 hours		
Care Plan	☐ initiated within 24 hours of admission ☐ problems selected specific to patient ☐ interventions specific to the patient ☐ goals listed ☐ evidence of problem resolution documented ☐ additions to care plan as condition changes		
Postpartum Education	☐ education documented on appropriate inpatient form/screens ☐ education methods correlate with patient's learning preferences ☐ patient's response to education documented		
Post-delivery Orders	☐ orders signed, dated and timed ☐ pre-printed orders initiated by an order ☐ STAT or now orders implemented within defined time frames ☐ other orders within time frame ☐ home medication addressed by physician		
Medication	☐ pain medications administered as ordered ☐ MAR free of unapproved abbreviations		
Pain Assessment and Reassessment	☐ conducted at frequency required by policy ☐ numerical score documented ☐ if analgesic given, reassessment done		
Discharge Instructions	☐ provided by physician ☐ signed by patient		
Initial Newborn Care	☐ list requirements ☐ ☐		
Newborn Orders	☐ orders obtained before non-nursing care initiated ☐ pre-printed orders are initiated by an order ☐ orders signed, dated and timed		
Newborn Nursing Assessment	☐ list requirements ☐ ☐ ☐		
Newborn Physician Exam	☐ Completed within ____ hours of birth ☐ list items that are to be included and may be missed		

CONFIDENTIAL

Appendix

Figure A.9 ■ OB Cesarean Section—Tracer Recording Form

Med Record # _____

Reviewer(s) _____ **Date** _____

TOPIC	FINDINGS: check items indicating compliance	Describe Non-compliance Issues	Staff Name(s) for Follow-up
Pre-op Education	☐ education documented on appropriate form		
H & P pre-surgical	☐ completed within 30 days of surgery or use of prenatal records ☐ includes an update on day of surgery		
Anesthesia Assessment ☐ N/A	☐ pre-anesthesia assessment present ☐ ASA score ☐ past anesthesia history ☐ lung assessment ☐ anesthesia plan ☐ airway assessment of class, neck, and teeth ☐ informed consent obtained by anesthesia staff		
Consents ☐ N/A	☐ informed consent obtained and documented by physician ☐ permit signed and dated by patient ☐ permit witnesses by signature, date and time		
Universal Protocol ☐ N/A	☐ pre-procedure verification ☐ time out documented		
Post-anesthesia Care Unit ☐ N/A	☐ pain assessment conducted ☐ reassessment after pain med given ☐ post anesthesia recovery score documented ☐ Vital signs recorded at policy frequency		
Immediate Postoperative/post-procedure Note ☐ N/A	☐ handwritten on chart ☐ hand written note includes: surgeon, assistants, procedure, description of procedure, findings, EBL, specimens and postoperative condition		
Post-anesthesia Visit	☐ performed by anesthesia provider ☐ entry signed, dated and timed ☐ performed after patient had recovered from anesthesia but before 48 hours of cesarean		

Page 1 of 1   CONFIDENTIAL

Additional Forms

Figure A.10 ■ Infection Control—Tracer Recording Form

Department _____ Med Rec# _____

Reviewer(s) _____ Date _____

Type of Infection _____

TOPIC	FINDINGS: check items indicating compliance	Describe Non-compliance Issues	Staff Name(s) for Follow-up
Identification of infection	☐ Notation in the record (location determined by organization) of the initiation of isolation or additional precautions ☐ Order for isolation obtained (if required by organization)		
Isolation Methods	☐ appropriate type selected for patient's infection ☐ appropriate signage on patient's door ☐ adequate supply of PPE available in cart outside patient's room		
Laboratory testing	☐ Initiation of precautions began immediately following the identification by lab testing results of a potential infectious disease		
Known patient	☐ The record was flagged with an infectious disease/carrier status ☐ N/A; No ID process exists ☐ Isolation/precautions were initiated immediately as documented in the record		
Inpatient Nursing Assessment	☐ If present on admission, assessment contains information related to the patients infection status		
Care Plan	☐ isolation/precautions entered on care plan ☐ initiated on day infection was identified ☐ a goal is listed		
Education	☐ education of patient documented regarding infectious disease ☐ education of patient documented regarding isolation practices ☐ education of family/visitors regarding isolation practices ☐ education methods correlate with patient's learning preferences		

Interview Questions

TOPIC	FINDINGS: check items indicating compliance	Describe Non-compliance Issues	Staff Name(s) for Follow-up
What reference is utilized to determine the type of isolation for the specified infection?	☐ to be completed by the organization; is this an unit manual, on-line document, etc.		

Page 1 of 2   CONFIDENTIAL

The Joint Commission Survey Coordinator's Handbook, 11th Edition

Appendix

Figure A.11 — Emergency Department—Tracer Recording Form

Med Rec# _____ Age _____

Reviewer(s) _____ Date _____

TOPIC	FINDINGS: check items indicating compliance	Describe Non-compliance Issues	Staff Name(s) for Follow-up
ED Triage Form	☐ presenting symptoms documented objectively ☐ triage level documented		
ED Physician Exam	☐ history & review of systems complete ☐ conclusions documented		
ED Nursing	☐ initial pain assessment documented ☐ pain medication ☐ pain reassessment ☐ appropriate pain scale for age & cognition ☐ abnormal vitals repeated		
ED Orders	☐ physician order for IV documented ☐ physician order for foley documented ☐ physician orders for medications documented ☐ orders free of unapproved abbreviations		
Pediatric Patient ☐ N/A	☐ Immunization status documented ☐ head circumference ≤ age 2		
Universal Protocol ☐ N/A	☐ pre-procedure verification ☐ site marking ☐ time out documented		
Medications	☐ home medication list compiled ☐ instructions regarding home medications provided to the patient at discharge ☐ list of home medications given to patient ☐ prescribed medications added to list		

Interview Questions

TOPIC	FINDINGS: check items indicating compliance	Describe Non-compliance Issues	Staff Name(s) for Follow-up
What is the process for obtaining and documenting a verbal order?	☐ physicians states the order, it is written down and then read back to the physician, he/she verifies it has been written down correctly and documented with VORB or TORB		
Name 4 of the unapproved abbreviations	☐ U ☐ IU ☐ QD ☐ QOD ☐ MS ☐ MSO₄ ☐ MgSO₄ ☐ HS ☐ trailing zero (2.0) ☐ lack of leading zero (.5)		

CONFIDENTIAL

Figure A.11 ■ Emergency Department—Tracer Recording Form (Cont.)

TOPIC	FINDINGS: check items indicating compliance	Describe Non-compliance Issues	Staff Name(s) for Follow-up
Describe how the Universal Protocol is used in this unit.	☐ Prior to an invasive or surgical procedure, patient identification is verified using the 2 identifiers ☐ Site is verified against the physician order, permit, x-rays, patient involvement and marked by nurse or physician performing the procedure ☐ Time out conducted with final verification of patient, procedure and site		
Name a pair of look-alike-sound-alike medications and the interventions implemented to decrease retrieval errors	☐ Add your organization's requirements ☐ ☐		
What medications have been identified as high risk? What practices have been implemented to decrease risk?	☐ labeled as high risk ☐ Add your organization's requirements ☐		
How is information regarding advance directives documented?	☐ Add your organization's requirements ☐ ☐		
What is occurring on your unit to improve quality?	☐ Answers may vary: core measures may be applicable		
Describe the patient handoff process and the information provided	☐ Add your organization's requirements ☐		
How has the goal regarding screening patients for risk of suicide been implemented?	☐ Add your organization's requirements		
Describe the organizations expectations for labeling medications and solutions on or off a sterile field.	☐ Labeling occurs even if there is only one medication being used ☐ Labeling occurs when any solution or medications is transferred from the original container to another container ☐ Labeled with: drug name, strength, amount, expiration date when not used within 24 hours and expiration time if expiration occurs < 24 hours ☐ No more than one medication or solution is labeled at one time ☐ Original container remain available ☐ Verification by two qualified individuals if preparer is not administering and if personnel relief occurs		
What data is being collected regarding patient flow?	☐ Add your organization's requirements ☐		

CONFIDENTIAL

Appendix

Figure A.12 ■ Resource Web Sites

Multidrug Resistant Organisms

http://www.cdc.gov/ncidod/dhqp/pdf/ar/mdroGuideline2006.pdf

http://www.ihi.org/IHI/Programs/Campaign/MRSAInfection.htm

http://www.wsha.org/files/82/HAI-ClostridiumDifficileStrategies.pdf

http://www.wsha.org/files/82/HAI-MRSAStrategies.pdf

http://www.cdc.gov/ncidod/dhqp/pdf/ar/mdroGuideline2006.pdf

Reducing Central Line Infections

http://www.ihi.org/IHI/Programs/Campaign/CentralLineInfection.htm

http://www.wsha.org/files/82/HAI-CentralLineStrategies.pdf

http://www.cdc.gov/nhsn/PDFs/pscManual/4PSC_CLABScurrent.pdf

Reducing Surgical Site Infections

http://www.ihi.org/IHI/Programs/Campaign/SSI.htm

http://www.wsha.org/files/82/HAI-SurgicalSiteStrategies.pdf

Getting Boards on Board

http://www.ihi.org/IHI/Programs/Campaign/BoardsonBoard.htm

Case Studies: Your Chance to Determine What Went Wrong

http://www.ihi.org/IHI/Programs/IHIOpenSchool/CaseStudies.htm

Figure A.12 ■ Resource Web Sites (Cont.)

Compendium of Strategies to Prevent Healthcare Associated Infections in Acute Care Hospitals

http://www.wsha.org/files/82/HAI-SummaryOfStrategies.pdf

Improving Patient Safety Through Infection Control: A New Healthcare Imperative

http://www.wsha.org/files/82/HAI-ImperativeOfPatientSafetyThroughInfectionControl.pdf

National Council of State Boards of Nursing

https://www.ncsbn.org/515.htm

National Boards of Respiratory Care

https://www.nbrc.org/StateLicensure/AgencyDirectory/tabid/54/Default.aspx

Radiology Technician State Contacts

https://www.arrt.org/

FREE HEALTHCARE COMPLIANCE AND MANAGEMENT RESOURCES!

Need to control expenses yet stay current with critical issues?

Get timely help with FREE e-mail newsletters from HCPro, Inc., the leader in healthcare compliance education. Offering numerous free electronic publications covering a wide variety of essential topics, you'll find just the right e-newsletter to help you stay current, informed, and effective. All you have to do is sign up!

With your FREE subscriptions, you'll also receive the following:

- Timely information, to be read when convenient with your schedule
- Expert analysis you can count on
- Focused and relevant commentary
- Tips to make your daily tasks easier

And here's the best part—there's no further obligation—just a complimentary resource to help you get through your daily challenges.

It's easy. Visit *www.hcmarketplace.com/free/e-newsletters* to register for as many free e-newsletters as you'd like, and let us do the rest.

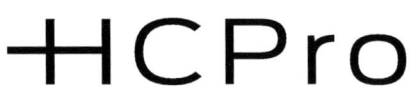

Insight for healthcare compliance and management